DOING RAPID QUALITATIVE RESEARCH

Sara Miller McCune founded SAGE Publishing in 1965 to support the dissemination of usable knowledge and educate a global community. SAGE publishes more than 1000 journals and over 800 new books each year, spanning a wide range of subject areas. Our growing selection of library products includes archives, data, case studies and video. SAGE remains majority owned by our founder and after her lifetime will become owned by a charitable trust that secures the company's continued independence.

Los Angeles | London | New Delhi | Singapore | Washington DC | Melbourne

CECILIA
VINDROLA-PADROS

DOING RAPID QUALITATIVE RESEARCH

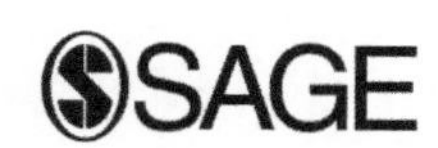

Los Angeles | London | New Delhi
Singapore | Washington DC | Melbourne

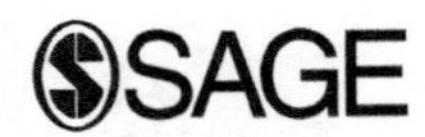

Los Angeles | London | New Delhi
Singapore | Washington DC | Melbourne

SAGE Publications Ltd
1 Oliver's Yard
55 City Road
London EC1Y 1SP

SAGE Publications Inc.
2455 Teller Road
Thousand Oaks, California 91320

SAGE Publications India Pvt Ltd
B 1/I 1 Mohan Cooperative Industrial Area
Mathura Road
New Delhi 110 044

SAGE Publications Asia-Pacific Pte Ltd
3 Church Street
#10-04 Samsung Hub
Singapore 049483

Editor: Alysha Owen
Senior assistant editor: Charlotte Bush
Production editor: Victoria Nicholas
Marketing manager: Ben Griffin-Sherwood
Cover design: Candice Harman
Typeset by: diacriTech
Printed in the UK

Library of Congress Control Number: 2020952153

British Library Cataloguing in Publication data

A catalogue record for this book is available from the British Library

ISBN 978-1-5264-9737-6
ISBN 978-1-5264-9736-9 (pbk)

To my beautiful Julian,
for teaching me to see the world in a different way.

TABLE OF CONTENTS

LIST OF TABLES

LIST OF FIGURES

1

INTRODUCTION

Many years ago, I was approached by a senior manager in a children's hospital who was looking for a research team to evaluate a new service he had implemented in the hospital. The purpose of the new service was to deliver some of the care required by patients as an outpatient service, reducing the need for children and their parents to be admitted to the hospital. A few months after the service had been rolled out, it was not providing care to the number of patients that had originally been estimated. This low number of patient cases was mainly due to staff members' unwillingness and inability to refer patients to the service.

I was asked to put together a team to carry out a diagnostic study to identify the main reasons why staff were not referring patients to the service. The caveat was that important decisions would need to be made about continuing or discontinuing the service at the next Board meeting. This meant findings would need to be delivered in two months. From my point of view, this meant I would need to assemble a team, design a study protocol, collect data, analyse it and disseminate it in a user-friendly way in less than eight weeks.

It was not an easy process, but we managed to carry out a rapid appraisal of the main barriers to referral. We carried out interviews with staff, observed referral processes and the delivery of care in the outpatients' area and conducted documentary analysis. We developed a visual summary of the findings (similar to an infographic) and shared them by the deadline. The Board decided to continue with the service provided that the service leads develop action plans to address each of the referral barriers we had identified in our evaluation. The main changes that needed to be made were the development of better educational materials for hospital staff in relation to the services the outpatient clinic could provide, the simplification of the paperwork required to refer patients (as some staff found this to be too time consuming) and the creation of a follow-up system where staff who referred patients to the outpatient service would be informed about these patients' outcomes after they were seen as outpatients. This was my first exposure to rapid qualitative research and, needless to say, I fell in love with this field.

We (by we I mean our research team that has recently become the Rapid Research Evaluation and Appraisal Lab [RREAL]) then went on to design and implement a wide range of rapid studies, including rapid ethnographies, rapid appraisals, rapid evaluations and rapid assessment procedures (RAPs). We reviewed the work others had done with these approaches (Johnson and Vindrola-Padros, 2017; Vindrola-Padros and Johnson, 2020; Vindrola-Padros and Vindrola-Padros, 2018; Vindrola-Padros et al., 2021) and sought ways to experiment with methods and advance the field of rapid qualitative research. We started being approached by other researchers, practitioners and students interested in the work and became aware of the need for formal training on these topics. We developed training courses for postgraduate students, clinicians, social scientists and managers, and it was at this point that we recognised the value of bringing together all of this information, our research experiences, previous studies, questions posed by our students, into one book.

The aim of the book is to develop capacity in the design, implementation, dissemination and use of findings generated through rapid qualitative research. I provide an overview of how these approaches have been used in the past, discuss the challenges of conducting rapid qualitative research through the use of real-world examples presented in the form of case studies and provide practical advice and guidelines for carrying out rapid and rigorous research. I also engage critically with this field, underscoring its main problems and limitations as well as situations when rapid approaches might not be suitable. I mainly focus on qualitative research but include examples of the collection and analysis of quantitative data, where relevant.

What Is Rapid Qualitative Research?

There is considerable debate in the field concerning the definition of rapid qualitative research. Beebe defined rapid qualitative inquiry (RQI) as 'intensive, team-based qualitative inquiry with a) a focus on the insider's or emic perspective, b) using multiple sources and triangulation, and c) using iterative data analysis and additional data collection to quickly develop a preliminary understanding of a situation' (2014: 3). McNall and Foster-Fishman (2007) sought to identify the common principles among all rapid evaluation and appraisal methods (REAMs) and concluded that the processes they had in common were:

- Rapid: Study lasted a few weeks or a few months.
- Participatory: Members from the community were involved in the design and implementation of the study.
- Team-based: Study was carried out by teams of researchers working collaboratively.
- Iterative: Data were analysed as they were collected in order to share emerging findings (McNall and Foster-Fishman, 2007: 159).

The study timeframes continue to be undefined, and what might be rapid for some is not rapid for others. For Scrimshaw and Hurtado (1987), for instance, rapid studies required anywhere from four to eight weeks. Handwerker (2001), however, argued that quick ethnographies required 90 days. According to Beebe (2014), rapid studies could be carried out in less than one month.

Qualitative research has also been defined in different ways, while some authors have focused on the type of data collected (i.e. data that cannot be quantified), others have argued that the distinguishing feature of qualitative research is its interpretive stance (Snape and Spencer, 2004). For the purpose of this book, I define rapid qualitative research as empirical research that focuses on documenting aspects of the world through the eyes of others, integrates the subjectivities of the researcher as part of the research process (i.e. reflexivity) and engages with some form of social theory (Flick, 2018; Lapan et al., 2011). Based on recent reviews that have sought to map the rapid research field, I consider rapid qualitative research to be qualitative research that lasts anywhere from a few days to six months (Johnson and Vindrola-Padros, 2017; Vindrola-Padros and Vindrola-Padros, 2018) or might have a longer timeframe, but include multiple short and intensive stages of data collection and analysis, as in the case of rapid feedback evaluations and rapid cycle evaluations (Vindrola-Padros et al., 2021).

What Are the Main Rapid Qualitative Research Approaches?

Rapid qualitative research has a long-standing history in the social sciences. Some authors have argued that rapid fieldwork techniques have been used consistently since at least the 1970s through quick surveys or sondeos used in rural anthropology (Chambers, 1994b). Organisations such as the World Health Organization (WHO) and the United Nations International Drug Control Programme (UNDCP) were responsible for developing initial attempts to speed up the delivery of findings (Fitch et al., 2000). This was initially done by anthropologists carrying out fieldwork on nutrition and primary care, who developed rapid methodologies such as RAPs (Scrimshaw and Hurtado, 1987). RAPs were developed to conduct rapid assessments of health-seeking behaviour by anthropologists or other professionals trained in field methods (Scrimshaw and Hurtado, 1984, 1987). These authors developed a RAP manual with data collection guides to complete fieldwork within a timeframe of four to eight weeks (Scrimshaw and Hurtado, 1987).

Other anthropologists developed approaches such as rapid ethnographic assessments (REAs) through a dietary management of diarrhoea programme led by Johns Hopkins University (Bentley et al., 1988). This approach was originally developed to provide quick assessments on local conditions to inform the design and implementation of interventions and obtain in-depth knowledge on local beliefs and attitudes (Bentley et al., 1988).

Rapid appraisals drew heavily from REAs and other forms of ethnographic and case study research. The main focus of rapid appraisals was on getting the insider's perspective, and this was achieved through the use of intensive teamwork for data collection and data analysis (where members of the community could form part of the team), and iterative data collection and analysis (Beebe, 1995, 2004). Researchers also experimented with more participatory approaches, involving community members in the research process (Chambers, 1994). The most emblematic participatory approach was participatory rural appraisal (PRA). Frequently associated with the work of Robert Chambers, PRA has been defined as 'a family of approaches and methods to enable rural people to share, enhance and analyse their knowledge of life and conditions, to plan and to act' (Chambers, 1994b: 953). It focused on the empowerment of local participants and involved data collection from a variety of sources (Rifkin, 1992).

Evaluators have also developed rapid approaches, including the development of rapid assessment methodology (RAM) in the 1990s for research focused on injecting drug use, rapid evaluation methods (REMs) and, more recently, rapid feedback evaluations and RCEs (to allow for longer evaluations, but with short cycles of data collection and analysis to share findings) (McNall et al., 2004; Shrank, 2013). These evaluations can be mixed methods, but a recent review has pointed to the frequent use of qualitative research designs (Vindrola-Padros et al., 2021).

Another recent trend has been an increase in the popularity of rapid ethnographies (Vindrola-Padros and Vindrola-Padros, 2018). Rapid ethnographies tend to have the following characteristics:

- The research is carried out over a short, compressed or intensive period of time.
- The research captures relevant social, cultural and behavioural information and focuses on human experiences and practices.
- The research engages with anthropological and other social science theories and promotes reflexivity.
- Data are collected from multiple sources and triangulated during analysis.
- More than one field researcher can be used to save time and cross-check data.
- Research designs and steps involved in the implementation of the study are reported clearly in publications and other forms of dissemination (Vindrola-Padros and Vindrola-Padros, 2018).

Rapid ethnographies have diversified and currently include quick ethnographies, focused ethnographies, focused rapid ethnographic evaluation (FREE), rapid ethnographies and short-term ethnographies. These approaches are normally used to capture in depth, rich data with targeted, intensive fieldwork (Knoblauch, 2005; Pink and Morgan, 2013). Chapter 3 provides a detailed overview of rapid ethnographies and the rapid qualitative research approaches mentioned earlier. An important thing to note is that, although these approaches share core features, their particular singularities provide researchers with a broad repertoire of approaches for carrying out rapid qualitative research, depending on preferences in relation to the degree of participatory research, structure and team-based work.

How Is Rapid Research Used and When Is It Useful?

There is variability in how rapid research has been used and it is important to go over different design approaches. Figure 1.1 presents the main types of rapid research use and integration with other types of studies we have found to date. Rapid research can be used

(1) as a preliminary study used to inform longer-term research (Coreil et al., 1989), (2) as a short study carried out to explore new questions that might have remained or emerged after the longer study ended (Munoz-Plaza et al., 2016), (3) in parallel to a longer study, potentially using rapid feedback loops or cycles to inform the development of the longer study (McNall et al., 2004; Shrank, 2013) or (4) as a study on its own (Beebe, 2001).

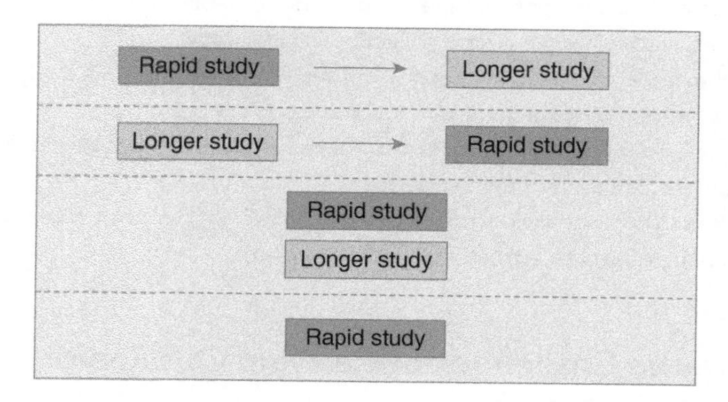

Figure 1.1 Common rapid/longer-term research designs

The use of rapid research is diverse and these types of studies tend to be flexible and easily adaptable to changing circumstances. However, this does not mean that rapid research is appropriate for all research contexts and topics. Nunns (2009) developed a resource–time matrix to examine the value of carrying out certain types of evaluations in the policy context. According to her, 'proper' evaluations were those where researchers had a higher level of resource and less time or a higher level of resource and more time (Nunns 2009). The former often involved evaluations where findings were time-critical for stakeholders, but researchers had a team at their disposal and used rapid research and evaluation methods. The latter involved evaluations that were not as constrained by time (or constrained in a different way, such as requiring regular feedback loops of findings), and more complex designs could used (Nunns, 2009).

Evaluations where researchers had more time but fewer resources might not be 'nice to do' as the lack of resources might imply they were not a priority for policymakers (Nunns, 2009). Evaluations with fewer resources and less time should only be carried out if the researchers had confidence in the quality of available data. If new data needed to be collected or the quality of the existing data was questionable, these should be avoided (Nunns, 2009).

The matrix developed by Nunns (2009) is not only useful for evaluations but for other types of projects as well. Factors such as the purpose of the study, type of research question, resources available, times when findings are required and data availability can determine the type of research design and can help researchers decide whether rapid research is the best option. Nunns' (2009) framework is also helpful for raising red flags in cases where low levels of resource and time pressures could lead to low-quality studies.

In our experience, there are a series of situations when it might be best to avoid carrying out rapid qualitative studies and these include:

- When the time and resources available for the study are severely constrained and there is a lack of existing evidence to help inform the study design
- When there are clear signs that the team will not be able to get access to the people or spaces required to carry out data collection for the study
- When the research questions cannot be answered with a rapid study design as they require long-term engagement with a specific topic or area
- When the findings of the study can produce negative consequences for some of the stakeholders (intended or unintended)
- When researchers are being asked to 'cut corners' or carry out research in a way that might violate quality or ethical standards of research

What Are the Challenges of Carrying Out Rapid Qualitative Research?

The development of rapid qualitative research approaches has not gone uncontested. Some authors have positioned themselves completely against this type of research, others have cautioned against their mainstream use (Fitch et al., 2000) and a third group has critically examined their design and implementation and tried to develop strategies to help overcome their challenges (Vindrola-Padros, 2020; Vindrola-Padros and Vindrola-Padros, 2018). I discuss the challenges of rapid qualitative research in greater depth in Chapter 6, but at this stage in the book, it is important to highlight that one of the main challenges faced by researchers using rapid qualitative research is overcoming the assumption that, when research is rapid, it will lose rigour and the richness and depth normally associated with qualitative research (Pink and Morgan, 2013). According to this assumption, building relationships with participants and getting a good understanding of complex social and cultural issues takes time (Beebe, 2001). In order to reach its full potential, qualitative research should not be carried out over short periods of time.

Proponents of rapid qualitative research have not disagreed completely with this assumption but have argued that there are different reasons why one would engage in rapid qualitative research, that these approaches might not be suitable for all topics and contexts and, more importantly, that there are ways of carrying out rapid qualitative research where rigour can still be maintained and rich data can still be generated. Robert Chambers, considered the father of PRA, argued that rapid approaches could be 'too over-sold, too rapidly adopted, badly done, and then discredited, to suffer an undeserved, premature burial as has occurred with other innovative research approaches' (Chambers, 1991). Beebe (2004) also urged researchers to distinguish between 'rapid' and 'rushed' research, alluding to commonly held assumptions that rapid research lacks rigour. According to them and several other authors, rapid qualitative approaches, when carried out properly, guarantee rigour without sacrificing speed (Fitch et al., 2000; Manderson and Aaby, 1992b).

Another related challenge lies in the theoretical grounding of rapid qualitative research that some researchers fear can be difficult to maintain due to time pressures and the fact that most rapid research is designed with the specific purpose to provide actionable findings. According to some authors, this 'applied' nature of rapid qualitative research can lead to the production of research that is instrumental, atheoretical and without a critical angle (Cupit et al., 2018; Manderson and Aaby, 1992a).

The tension between the breadth and depth of data has also been identified as problematic in rapid qualitative research (Bentley et al., 1988; Manderson and Aaby, 1992b). One recurrent concern is that rapid qualitative research will not be able to capture all of the relevant social, cultural, political and economic factors at stake and it will not be able to engage with conflicting views or contradictions. As a result, the depth and focus on complexity that makes qualitative research unique will be lost. As is the case of all research, the production of knowledge through rapid qualitative research approaches will be partial. As Manderson and Aaby have indicated, 'any research done within a short time frame is necessarily circumscribed, and its strength is the focusing that occurs as a consequence of this' (1992a: 845).

Rapid qualitative researchers have developed a series of techniques to make sure their studies can engage with the most salient issues and capture, at least to some extent, a wide range of views. They have also tried to promote transparency and detailed reporting of study designs to indicate which areas have been covered in depth throughout the study and which might have been glossed over (Utarini et al., 2001). An important factor to consider is that gaps in data collection could be a matter of study design, regardless of the length of the study (i.e. long studies also deal with tensions between breadth and depth). In Chapter 3, I discuss the steps researchers can take to try to address these potential issues, including the development of preparatory work to focus the research questions and inform the study design.

Related to concerns around not capturing contradictions and conflicting views are issues of sampling in rapid qualitative research. Time pressures might mean that researchers recruit participants or observe situations that are easily accessible. This might mean that the views of some participants will feature more prominently in the study and a multiplicity of voices will be lost (Harris et al., 1997). Rapid qualitative researchers have tried to address this potential challenge through the careful design of sampling guides (sometimes called sampling frameworks or briefs), where researchers map the different groups of participants they would like to include in the study (for instance, based on gender, age, occupation) and set out sampling targets for each (Handwerker, 2001). During the study, they would attempt to recruit participants from the different groups deemed important for the study. I describe different sampling techniques in Chapter 4.

In a recent review on the use of rapid ethnographies in healthcare, we found that not enough attention was paid by researchers to reflexivity. By reflexivity, we meant 'the author's critical analysis of the position they occupy throughout the research process and how they participate in the production of knowledge' (Vindrola-Padros and Vindrola-Padros, 2018: 7). We argued that this represented a significant limitation for this type of research as the researcher's critical account of their 'self-location', interests, pre-assumptions and life experiences always shapes the research process, but authors were not discussing this openly in their papers. Even though this challenge is not limited to rapid research, it is an ongoing challenge in rapid qualitative research that we will revisit in the book and will engage with in depth in Chapters 2 and 7.

Book Outline

This book is designed as an introductory aid to rapid qualitative research. It is broad enough to cover most rapid research approaches, tools and problems, but it also provides in-depth discussions of the common challenges and strategies used while carrying out this type of work. It contains discussion questions, case studies and exercises for use in a classroom environment, but these are also designed to be useful for self-guided work. The book can be used in its entirety and followed from beginning to end, as it walks through all the stages of research (study design, implementation and dissemination). The chapters are also written as standalone chapters, so these can be selected and used at different time points and in different order.

The introductory chapter presents an overview of rapid qualitative research, its main uses and challenges, and it sets out the aims of the book and its overall structure.

Chapter 2 provides a brief historical overview of a wide range of rapid methods including rapid appraisals, RAPs, rapid rural appraisal (RRA), PRA, REA, RQI, the rapid assessment, response and evaluation model (RARE), rapid evaluations, rapid ethnography, quick ethnography, focused ethnography and short-term ethnography. The chapter follows Beebe's (1995) definition of rapid appraisals, which conceptualises this approach as 'the production of quick results and the simultaneous use of research techniques associated with three concepts: 1) a system perspective, 2) triangulation of data collection, and 3) iterative collection and analysis'. It includes a brief history of rapid appraisals (for instance their frequent use in public health initiatives) and describes their relationships with other types of rapid research approaches (i.e. RAPs). The work of Bentley et al. (1988) is used to demonstrate how REAs were carried out in practice. The chapter discusses more recent developments of rapid ethnographies: quick ethnographies proposed by Handwerker (2001), focused ethnographies proposed by Knoblauch (2005) and short-term ethnographies proposed by Pink and Morgan (2013). This chapter draws from McNall and Foster-Fishman's (2007) classification of REAMs to present the reader with an overview of rapid evaluation designs. Four main types of rapid evaluations are presented: real-time evaluation (RTE), REMs, rapid cycle evaluation (RCE), and rapid feedback evaluation (RFE).

Chapter 3 is the main chapter addressing the stage of design. It discusses the preliminary work that can be carried out to inform the research questions guiding a study and its design. The chapter introduces the concept of a 'scoping phase', which is normally used to engage relevant stakeholders in the design of the rapid study, to make sure the research questions are relevant and the sharing of findings is carried out in a timely way. I present strategies for selecting the methods for data collection and analysis, developing the sampling strategy and dissemination plan.

Chapter 4 includes a step-by-step guide for carrying out data collection in rapid qualitative studies. The chapter also provides information on how these steps vary according to the types of design presented in Chapter 3. The chapter includes descriptions of methods for data collection, such as interviews, focus groups, observations, mapping and visual methods (photovoice, film and drawings). Emphasis is placed on the adaptations that can be made to these methods to enable rapid data collection. Examples from published studies are used to demonstrate how these adaptations were made in practice. The chapter also includes practical tools for facilitating team-based interviews and observations, process mapping and the writing of fieldnotes.

Chapter 5 focuses on describing data analysis approaches commonly used in qualitative research: content analysis, thematic analysis and framework analysis. The chapter includes strategies for reducing the amount of time required for data analysis, such as the use of RAP sheets, selected transcription of interview recordings, analysis directly from audio recordings and mind mapping during focus groups. The chapter includes examples of analytical frameworks.

A series of challenges have been identified in rapid research, which are mainly produced by time pressures, the reliance on teams of field researchers, the instrumental or pragmatic nature of some rapid designs (which might jeopardise the independence of the research) and the lack of attention paid to theory and reflexivity. As a consequence, rapid research is often thought of being 'quick and dirty'. *Chapter 6* explores challenges such as (1) conducting rigorous research without sacrificing speed, (2) ensuring teams of researchers collect and analyse data in a standardised way, (3) developing reflexive research practices and (4) the funding and sustainability of rapid research teams. The chapter includes a discussion of ethical governance processes, arguing that, even though studies must be carried out quickly, the same ethical principles as those of long-term studies must be followed (i.e. informed consent, do no harm, confidentiality and anonymity). It also presents a few strategies for streamlining the review of applications for ethical approval, showing examples of ethical review committees around the world that have established quicker and simpler review processes for studies that are low risk and time-sensitive.

All rapid research approaches presented in this book were developed to produce 'actionable findings', that is, findings that can be used to make changes in policy and/or practice. However, there is limited knowledge on how findings are normally disseminated in rapid research, and, even less, on how these findings are used. *Chapter 7* outlines the strategies that can be used throughout all stages of the research to maximise its impact. It highlights the importance of developing groups of stakeholders who can act in an advisory capacity throughout the study, ensuring the study is relevant but also facilitating the incorporation of findings into changes in practice. The chapter also proposes the establishment of regular feedback loops, where findings from the study are shared on a continuous basis and not only after the study has ended. The frequency and format of feedback are discussed and the chapter proposes alternatives for sharing information (i.e. traditional written reports, infographics, videos, podcasts).

Chapter 8 provides a case study of a rapid qualitative study by describing the life cycle of a rapid appraisal carried out during the COVID-19 pandemic. It includes a month-by-month description of the implementation of the study, describing the challenges we faced and how we addressed them. It mentions issues with sampling, team composition and coordination, the training of researchers and dissemination. *Chapter 9* describes an additional case study, one that describes the design of a rapid evaluation aimed at exploring the implementation of a participatory programme to support parents of children with learning disabilities.

Chapter 10 provides an overview of current gaps and limitations in the ways in which rapid research is used today. This chapter presents a description of new developments in this field as well as future areas of research.

Recommendations for Using the Exercises in the Book

Most chapters of the book include exercises. The exercises were designed with two goals in mind. If the book is to be used in a course on rapid qualitative research, my recommendation is to use the book in sequential order and have students work through the exercises as each chapter is read and discussed. The exercises walk students through the different stages of rapid qualitative research, helping them to design and implement their own studies. Alternatively, if only sections of the book are used in the course, some exercises can be selected to exemplify specific topics (i.e. aspects of data collection or dissemination).

I wrote this book after teaching an intensive course on rapid qualitative research to postgraduate students for several years. In the course, I presented the topics included in the book (in the same order as laid out in the book), we worked through the exercises in pairs and then as a group and the students then applied what they learned in class to their own projects. Most students were working either on a dissertation or a thesis, so the aim was for them to use the course to finalise their research designs and plan the implementation of the study. After working independently, they would return to class and share with classmates how they had applied the learning from the previous class to their own studies (this was done before introducing a new topic). This process of sharing represented a great opportunity for peer-to-peer learning.

If the book is used to design and implement a study, then option A exercises will be more appropriate. The option A exercises are designed to take a study topic from a research idea to full-study protocol. The book, however, is also designed for readers who might not have any exposure to research and will not have a specific study topic in mind. In this case, the exercises labelled as option B include examples of studies (either my own research or published studies) that can be used to work through the exercises. Experienced rapid qualitative researchers might want to jump around the book and pay closer attention to some of the newer techniques or areas where they are encountering problems.

Chapter Summary

- Rapid qualitative research can be defined as empirical research that focuses on documenting aspects of the world through the eyes of others, integrates the subjectivities of the researcher as part of the research process (i.e. reflexivity), engages with some form of social theory and has a duration of a few days to six months.
- Rapid qualitative research has a long-standing history and multiple approaches exist, including rapid appraisals, RAPs, RRA, RARE, rapid evaluations and rapid ethnographies, among others.
- Rapid qualitative research can be used as a study on its own or can be connected to a longer study.
- Factors such as the purpose of the study, type of research question, available resources, times when findings are required and data availability can determine the type of research design and can help researchers decide whether rapid research is the best option.
- Researchers carrying out rapid qualitative research face challenges in relation to perceptions about the quality of the study, validity of the data, credibility and perceived rigour.
- Researchers have developed a series of strategies for the design of research questions, sampling, theoretical engagement, reporting and dissemination of findings to address these challenges.

Discussion Questions

1. Pick one of the challenges of doing rapid qualitative research described in the chapter. How would you address this challenge in your own research?
2. Are there any challenges of rapid qualitative research missing from the chapter?
3. When should we avoid using rapid qualitative research designs ?

Exercise 1

Is My Study Suitable for Rapid Research?

In this chapter, I have discussed the main challenges of carrying out rapid qualitative research, situations when these approaches might be useful and situations when they should be avoided.

Option A

Think about your own study and develop a table like the following. In the first column, list the reasons why you think this study is suitable for rapid qualitative research. In the second column, list any doubts you might have about the study's suitability for rapid qualitative research. In the last column, list any challenges you anticipate in the design and implementation of the study.

A	B	C
Reasons why this could be rapid qualitative research	Doubts about suitability as a rapid qualitative study	Potential challenges

Now that you have created the table, reflect on the following questions:

1. When you look at the table, do the reasons listed in column A outweigh the doubts in column B?
2. Is there an overlap between the doubts listed in column B and the potential challenges you identified in column C?
3. Look at the potential challenges you listed in column C. What are some of the strategies you could use to address these? Can you reduce the impact of these challenges by designing your study in a different way?

Option B

Read the following brief description of the study.

School leaders noticed an increase in the number of children transferring to the school from areas that were not in its normal catchment area. These 'travelling' children were identified as having lower levels of attainment than the other children at the school and a higher level of social care needs. In order to identify the needs of incoming children and adapt their learning plans accordingly, the school headteacher contacted your team to carry out a rapid study focused on documenting children's (and their families') needs and experiences.

The research team had four part-time researchers with expertise in qualitative and quantitative research. The school was not sure about the quality of its routinely collected data. Findings were required within a two-month timeframe to inform decisions regarding the adaptation of learning plans, but the study could be longer and additional findings shared at a later date.

Develop a table like the following one. In the first column, list the reasons why you think this study is suitable for a rapid qualitative research approach. In the second column, list any doubts you might have about the study's suitability for rapid qualitative research. In the last column, list any challenges you anticipate in the design and implementation of the study.

A	B	C
Reasons why this could be rapid qualitative research	Doubts about suitability as a rapid qualitative study	Potential challenges

Now that you have created the table, reflect on the following questions:

1. When you look at the table, do the reasons listed in column A outweigh the doubts in column B?
2. Is there an overlap between the doubts listed in column B and the potential challenges you identified in column C?
3. Look at the potential challenges you listed in column C. What are some of the strategies the researchers could use to address these? Can they reduce the impact of these challenges by designing their study in a particular way?

2

A BRIEF OVERVIEW OF RAPID QUALITATIVE RESEARCH APPROACHES

Rapid qualitative research is not new; it encompasses a wide range of research approaches developed as early as the 1970s. These approaches have changed, cross-fertilised and generated completely new ways of doing qualitative research over short periods of time. In this chapter, I try to reconstruct this history of rapid qualitative research and provide an overview of over 15 approaches that have been used to date. I also flag some recent methodological developments that could become popular rapid qualitative research approaches in the near future.

Rapid Rural Appraisal

Heywood (1990: 46) defined rapid rural appraisals (RRAs) as 'a strategy for appraising a particular situation in the most cost-effective manner possible with appropriate levels of timeliness, accuracy and relevance'. RRAs depended on multidisciplinary teams, the combination of different sources of data and the use of local knowledge and expertise. These are one of the oldest rapid qualitative research approaches, emerging in the late 1970s (Manderson and Aaby, 1992a). RRAs were pragmatic as they emphasised existing data, use of research teams with a high level of expertise and research skills, a mixture of qualitative research methods and the involvement of local community members in the research process. Chambers described data collection in RRAs as focusing on what was 'relevant, timely and usable' (1981: 95).

Participatory Rural Appraisal

Chambers added a slightly more participatory twist to RRAs and contributed to the development of participatory rural appraisals (PRAs). According to him, PRAs emerged out of the recognition that local community members could make contributions to research and could be empowered to lead on their own appraisals (Chambers, 2008). In many of these appraisals, the research was carried out internally and outsiders were only brought in during analysis or even dissemination stages (Chambers and Blackburn, 1996). When comparing RRAs and PRAs, Chambers (1994) indicated that RRAs were more verbal and active with outsiders in the sense that the main objective was data collection by outsiders. PRAs were more visual and active with locals, and had a sharing-empowering approach where the objectives were evaluation, learning, action and monitoring by insiders (Chambers, 1994).

Rapid Ethnographic Assessment

In the late 1980s, anthropologists began to question the amount of time required in the field to collect information on health beliefs and practices. Bentley argued that 'anthropologists with long-term experience in applied health care research and planning have become convinced that the process of gathering essential ethnographic data can be a relatively rapid process, and is indeed a necessary response to programmatic time and budgetary constraints' (1988: 107). These authors believed that detailed ethnographic data could not be collected rapidly, but the basic information required to inform health programme delivery could (Bentley et al., 1988).

Rapid ethnographic assessments (REAs) were defined as 'a methodological approach that is intended to maximise the strengths of the anthropological, open-ended approach to data gathering, in a manner that permits data to be utilised in multi-staged research' (Bentley et al., 1988: 108). According to McNall and Foster-Fishman (2007), REAs were different from other approaches such as PRAs and rapid appraisals because they used a more limited range of research methods and focused more on exploring participants' worldview and their perceptions of health issues.

One defining characteristic of REAs was the development of structured field guides. Field guides provided guidelines for the type of information required to inform health programme delivery. The first guides were developed by Bentley et al. (1988) to collect data on the beliefs and practices related to diarrhoea in children, infant feeding practices, healthcare utilisation, child care patterns and family work roles (see Table 2.1).

Table 2.1 Example of field guide developed by Bentley et al. (1988) to explore dietary management of diarrhoea in Peru

I. Introduction
   a. Purpose of the project
   b. Purpose of the use of ethnographic guide
   c. Field ethics and interview methods
II. Background site information
   a. Collection of secondary data
   b. Description of ecological, socio-cultural, political site
   c. Food production, availability, preparation
   d. Women's work roles and time allocation

III. Selection of field sites and informants
   a. Rough demographic mapping
   b. Identification of key informants
   c. Identification of non-key informants
IV. Illness taxonomies
   a. Illnesses commonly experienced: Names, symptoms, causes, consequences
   b. Child illnesses: Names, symptoms, causes, consequences
   c. Diarrhoea: How does it fit into larger illness taxonomy
V. Diarrhoea-building a 'folk taxonomy' of diarrhoea
   a. General beliefs about diarrhoea
   b. Names of each diarrhoea type
   c. Definitions, symptoms, causes, consequences and treatments of each diarrhoea type
   d. Developmental sequence of episode by diarrhoea 'type'
VI. Child feeding
   a. Normal feeding patterns
      1. Beliefs about child feeding
      2. Weaning foods
         a. Age of introduction
         b. Preparation
   b. Feeding during/after diarrhoea
      1. General beliefs about feeding during diarrhoea
      2. Foods to be avoided (list, reasons)
      3. 'Special' foods to be given (list, reasons)
      4. Variation by diarrhoea 'type'
      5. Variations in feeding during stages of illness, convalescence
VII. 'The last diarrhoea episode'
   a. Description of episode: When, who, why (perceived cause), symptoms, treatments given, feeding during diarrhoea, outcome of episode
VIII. Analysis of data and report writing

REAs also depended on the recruitment of individuals familiar with the local culture/area to act as researchers. In their application of REAs in Nigeria and Peru, however, Bentley et al. (1988) outlined the difficulties of recruiting local researchers with the required skills to carry out the study or who might be available to work on the project at short notice. Furthermore, not all researchers could move around or relocate to the places where data needed to be collected (Bentley et al., 1988).

REAs have been developed to explore breastfeeding practices in Mexico (Guerrero et al., 1999), beliefs surrounding acute respiratory infections in children (Kresno et al., 1993), family planning practices among people living with HIV/AIDS in Nigeria (Garko, 2007), local attitudes and perceptions towards malaria in Zambia (Williams et al., 1999; see Table 2.2), diagnosis and management of fever in Ghana (Agyepong & Manderson, 1994), perceptions of childbirth and maternity services (Culhane-Pera et al., 2015), healthcare-seeking practices for ill children in Sierra Leone (Scott et al., 2014), perceptions of stroke-like symptoms (Hundt et al., 2004), perceptions of palliative care barriers and facilitators (Goepp et al., 2008), factors influencing antiretroviral therapy use in Thailand (Murray et al., 2016) and caregiver perspectives and experiences accessing childhood illness services (Shaw et al., 2016).

Table 2.2 Rapid ethnographic assessment of community perspectives of the efficacy of malaria treatment in Zambia (Williams et al., 1999)

Aim of the study: This study explored parents' acceptance of a new drug introduced by the Zambia Ministry of Health as a second-line antimalarial in Lundazi District. The authors carried out a rapid community ethnographic assessment to examine local attitudes and perceptions towards malaria and perceived efficacy of the new drug.

Data collection methods:

1. Focus group (FG) discussions (total of 16, 9 with mothers and 7 with fathers of children under 5)
2. In-depth interviews (36 in total, 8 with parents, 4 with drug vendors, 9 with traditional healers and 10 with facility-based health workers)
3. Free pile sorts and ranking on the 14 most salient traditional and modern malaria treatments

Study scope and duration: Data collection was carried out in eight communities and lasted one month.

Research team: The fieldwork was carried out by six school teachers from the Lundazi District who were recruited and trained in qualitative data collection by the research team. The interviews and FGs were carried out in the local language. The researchers audio recorded the FGs and interviews and documented their observations during these in the form of fieldnotes.

Data synthesis and analysis: Specific data analysis methods were not reported, but the authors indicated that members of the research team produced in-depth debriefings with field staff at the end of each day of data collection. These debriefings were used to expand the depth of the notes, verify interpretations of the data and ensure linguistic consistency.

Dissemination and use of findings: The authors used the findings to make recommendations on information, education and communication activities and health worker training for the new drug.

Reflections of the research team:

- It was helpful to use different methods to increase the accuracy of the data, including daily debriefing sessions with the field workers at the end of data collection, the presence of two researchers during each interview (one to do the interview and one to record notes) and translation and back-translation of study instruments.
- Enrolment for the study was slower than other previous studies in this area and this could be due to the fact that the study started at the end of the transmission season.
- The REA highlighted the need for an understanding of local perceptions of malaria, as proposed control activities might not be accepted by community members.

Rapid Appraisals and Rapid Assessments

Rapid assessments or appraisals also stemmed from anthropological research and were designed to obtain rich data on particular contexts rapidly, pragmatically and in a manner that was deemed more cost-effective (Vincent et al., 2000). Teams of researchers were used to collect data from key contacts or informants in the communities. These interviews were combined with other methods such as focus groups, community walks and mapping and surveys (Garrett & Downen, 2002). When possible, researchers used existing data sources and only collected new data if necessary (Aral et al., 2005). Even though rapid appraisals were flexible enough to be used for multiple research and evaluation purposes, they were normally used as diagnostic tools or to capture information from a particular community or specific topic that could then be used to design health programmes or interventions (Desmond et al., 2005; Kirsch, 1995; Trotter and Singer, 2005).

Rapid Assessment Procedures

Rapid assessment procedures (RAPs) were developed by anthropologists to improve health programme planning and evaluation by capturing the social and cultural factors that frame health behaviours (Fitch et al., 2000). According to Utarini et al. (2001), the term *rapid* emphasised the short amount of time for field data collection, *assessment* drew attention to a limited or focused scope of information for evaluation purposes and *procedures* indicated the use of a variety of formalised means of data collection. Time constraints and the high costs associated with long-term research were some of the main drivers of the development of this approach (Utarini et al., 2001). Furthermore, researchers believed that community members could make important contributions to the design and implementation of studies and should be a part of research teams (Harris et al., 1997). The distinguishing features of RAPs were:

- Formation of a multidisciplinary research team including a member from the cultural group of interest
- Development of materials to train team members
- Use of several data collection methods to verify information through triangulation
- Iterative data collection and analysis to facilitate continuous adjustment
- Completion of the project quickly, usually in four to six weeks (Harris et al., 1997)

One key aspect of RAPs was the belief that the methodology needed to be available to researchers outside of the social sciences and with no prior research experience (Manderson and Aaby, 1992a). RAP manuals were developed to guide researchers without a background in disease-based research skills or qualitative research (Fitch et al., 2000). The first manual was published by Scrimshaw and Hurtado in 1987 for their work on primary care and nutrition for UNICEF. It included 31 data collection guides covering topics such as characteristics of the community, household and primary healthcare providers (Scrimshaw and Hurtado, 1987) (see full list of topics in Table 2.3).

In addition to the limitations identified for rapid qualitative research in general, one limitation associated mainly with RAPs was the fear that important information might be missing as a result of its structured approach to data collection (for instance, through the use of pre-established manuals) (Manderson and Aaby, 1992b). Researchers expressed concern that RAP methodology left little room for serendipity during fieldwork and limited the capacity of researchers to make changes in the study design along the way (Manderson and Aaby, 1992b). Due to its reliance on the use of community members or individuals from the area/sector in question (normally with limited skills in research), potential issues with the quality of the data, and reliability of the study, have also been highlighted (Harris et al., 1997; Manderson and Aaby, 1992a).

Table 2.3 List of topics and methods covered in the rapid assessment procedure (RAP) manual data collection guides developed by Scrimshaw and Hurtado (1987)

Area	Method	Description
Community		
C. 1 Geographic characteristics	Documentary analysis, observations	
C. 2 Demographic and epidemiologic characteristics	Documentary analysis, interviews, observations	
C. 3 Socio-economic characteristics	Documentary analysis, interviews, observations	
C. 4 Overview of health resources	Interviews, observations	
Household		
H. 1 Household composition	Interviews	
H. 2 Household conditions	Interviews, observations	
H. 3 Socio-economic status	Interviews, informal conversations	Employment, land owned/rented, land cultivated, food stored, food sold, dependents
H. 4 Definitions of health and illness	Interviews, informal conversations	
H. 5 Common illnesses in children and possible treatments	Interviews, informal conversations, observations	Knowledge of illness, gravity, remedies or treatments, expenses, prevention
H. 6 Foods eaten by mothers and children	Interviews, observations	
H. 7 Diet and sick children	Interviews, informal conversations and observations	
H. 8 Morbidity history of adult family members	Interviews	List of illnesses in the past two weeks
H. 9 Morbidity history of children 5 years of age and under	Interviews	List of illnesses in the past two weeks and during the course of the study
H. 10 Inventory of household remedies	Interviews, observations	Use, origin, cost and purpose

Area	Method	Description
H. 11 History of most recent pregnancies and deliveries	Interviews	
H. 12 Use of health resources	Interviews	
H. 13 Use and experiences with official health resources	Interview/informal conversations	
Primary healthcare providers		
P. 1 Interview with head of community health service	Interview	Schedule, services offered, personnel, equipment, cost of services and medicines to patients, methods of payment, utilisation
P. 2 Interview with health staff	Interview	Interview with each staff member in the community health service
P. 3 Physical characteristics of health resource	Observation	Make a map and draw the route the patient follows. Describe the environment, including any visual or educational aids
P. 4 The waiting room	Observation	Number of patients waiting and under what conditions, length of time they wait, activities that take place while patients wait, interaction between staff and patients, positive and negative aspects of the environment
P. 5 The consultation	Observation	Sequence of events, interactions, explanation and instructions given to the patient
P. 6 Food distribution and/or anthropometric examination	Observation	Describe the complimentary food distribution programme and the anthropometric assessment
P. 7 Summary of user visit to health resource	Observation	Summarise the user's visit to the health resource by recording information in a table
P. 8 Pharmacies and stores selling pharmacies	Interview	Interview the owner or manager at each pharmacy store
P. 9 Pharmacy staff	Interview	Interview staff members at stores that sell medicines
P. 10 Exit interview	Interview	Interview patients as they leave the health resource

(Continued)

Table 2.3 (Continued)

Area	Method	Description
P. 11 Knowledge of diarrhoea and oral rehydration	Interview	Interview each staff member charged with the duties of primary care
P. 12 Preparation of oral solution	Observation	If there are packets of oral rehydration salts, observe the preparation of the solutions
P. 13 Growth monitoring and immunisation	Interview	Interview each staff member responsible for growth monitoring and/or immunisation
P. 14 Provider–patient interaction	Observation	

Studies using a RAP approach have covered a wide range of topics and generated the following manuals: the evaluation of primary care and nutrition programmes (Scrimshaw and Hurtado, 1987), epilepsy (Long et al., 1988), HIV/AIDS (Scrimshaw et al., 1991), the assessment of women's health (Gittelsohn, 1998), malaria (Agyepong et al., 1995) and household management of diarrhoea (Herman and Bentley, 1993). More recent studies using RAPs have looked at planning emergency services for children (Goepp et al., 2004) and clinical decision support systems (Ash et al., 2010, 2012; Wright et al., 2015). Utarini et al. (2001) have highlighted issues with the reporting of information in RAPs and have proposed 11 criteria for appraising studies using this design (see Chapter 6).

Rapid Assessment, Response and Evaluation

Rapid assessment, response and evaluation (RARE) was slightly different to some of the other approaches discussed so far in the sense that members of the community/area where the study took place normally identified the need for research or evaluation (Needle et al. 2003). In 1999, the Office of Public Health and Science in the United States developed a series of crisis response teams capable of providing training in RARE methodologies to communities affected by HIV/AIDS (Needle et al., 2003). In order for RARE projects to begin, local officials needed to contact the Office requesting assistance. The research team based in the Office of HIV/AIDS Policy met with the local officials to review potential design options, helped put together a local working group and assigned a field research team to help facilitate the assessment. The key RARE methodological assumptions identified to date include:

- ***Speed:*** Its duration is eight to ten weeks.
- ***Non-duplicative:*** It complements ongoing processes rather than replaces them.

- ***Triangulation:*** The use of multiple methods and multiple data sources increases the validity of the results.
- ***Focus on contexts and situations:*** It provides the opportunity to fit solutions into the local context, with cultural competency and accommodation of local values and conditions.
- ***Local involvement and community consultation:*** It can be conducted and owned at a local level.
- ***Pragmatic:*** It is designed to be highly targeted (it does not do everything for everyone) and produces practical adaptable intervention recommendations that are correct for local conditions.
- ***Evaluation:*** It includes a necessary evaluation component to determine the effectiveness of both RARE and the recommended interventions (Trotter et al., 2001).

The field research team was normally led by an ethnographer and the project included an intensive training programme for the local working group with the aim of generating local research capacity (Needle et al., 2003). The use of a structured programme for the training of local researchers was one of the key contributions of RARE to rapid qualitative research. Table 2.4 has an example of a three-day researcher training programme described by Brown et al. (2008).

RARE studies tended to combine focus groups, key informant interviews, observations, mapping and rapid 'street intercept' assessment interviews (Needle et al., 2003).

Table 2.4 Training of community members as field researchers based on Brown et al. (2008)

Day 1 of training

- Reviewed rapid assessment, response and evaluation (RARE) methods
- Reviewed study focused on health disparities, access to care, the health system and cultural factors
- Discussed community involvement in the field team (cultural guides) and advisory committee
- Discussed the triangulation of observations by cultural guides, experienced ethnographers and students, providing both 'nuance' and 'fresh eyes'
- Reviewed plan to begin with mapping and observation, then interviews, then focus groups and surveys
- Reviewed mixed-methods with triangulation of ethnographic data with epidemiology and administrative data linked to chart audits
- Discussed the purpose of ethnographic investigation: 'To define the extent of the cultural complex'
- Discussed lessons learned in prior rapid assessments
- Discussed inductive approach to identify emergent concepts (i.e. issues that arise through the study, rather than those defined in advance)
- Conducted fieldnote exercise: Team made fieldnotes of food-gathering behaviour at local food court and discussed the fact that fieldnotes should be descriptive and not interpretive. Examples of proper note-taking were described

(Continued)

Table 2.4 (Continued)

Day 2 of training

- Interview training: Techniques meant to elicit discursive answers, recognising and dealing with obstacles during the interview process
- Developed interview guide for community members and patients
- Homework to develop interview guide for staff
- 'Ethnographic expedition' exercise

Day 3 of training (delivered six days after day 2)

- Trainees worked together to revise questionnaire
- Debate over the use of 'cultural bias' and 'poor' in the questionnaire
- Focus group training: Elicit discursive answers, understand group consensus, ensure all voices are heard
- Focus group exercise to explain the paramount role of the moderator, when to intervene, how to address the group
- Discussed multiple topics that can arise in a live focus group
- Discussed human participant protection and research ethics
- Team identified potential community advisory board members to contact

RARE manuals and procedures for data collection are available and can be adapted to different contexts and topics (Trotter et al., 2001). Local working groups played a central role in the design and implementation of the study. They helped review available local data (surveillance, epidemiological, planning data, maps) and identify areas or at-risk groups (Brown et al., 2008). As mentioned before, members from the community/area where the study took place also participated in data collection and analysis. Research teams (composed of the field research teams and community members) met regularly to report on data collection and discuss emerging themes. Findings were also shared regularly with key stakeholders throughout the project. In a study of health disparities in urban disadvantaged communities in Florida, Brown et al. (2008) shared emerging findings with a local group of stakeholders on three occasions over a six-week period (at Week 1, Week 3 and Week 6).

Rapid Qualitative Inquiry

Although his earlier work focused on the development of rapid appraisal methods (Beebe, 1995), Beebe expanded his portfolio to include rapid assessment processes and, more recently, rapid qualitative inquiry (RQI) (Beebe, 2001, 2004, 2014). Rapid assessment process (not to be confused with RAP earlier) was based on two main concepts:

1 Intensive teamwork as part of the triangulation of data collection.
2 Intensive teamwork during the iterative process of data analysis and additional data collection (Beebe, 2001: 7).

In rapid assessment process and RQI, more than one researcher was always required for data collection and analysis (Beebe, 2014). At least two individuals needed to gain sufficient understanding of a situation over a short amount of time (normally one to six weeks), and by collecting data as a team, the interaction of team members added layers of interpretation to the research process (Beebe, 2001, 2014). For instance, when using these approaches, the team of researchers carried out interviews together. By having at least two members of the team present at each interview, they were able to capture different aspects of the conversation or follow up on different topics. The same could be expected when multiple people carried out observations together (Beebe, 2014).

Triangulation occurred when combining the data produced through different methods, but in the case of rapid assessment process, triangulation was also produced by the interaction of team members during data collection (Beebe, 2014). The assumption was that each team member contributed their own perceptions, theories, methods and academic disciplines, which led to the generation of a unique worldview and different ways of collecting and interpreting data (Beebe, 2001).

Another distinguishing feature of RQI and rapid assessment process was their emphasis on iterative data collection and analysis (Beebe, 2001, 2014). Data were analysed as researchers were collecting data, allowing the nearly real-time sharing of findings, but also pointing to gaps in data collection researchers could address before the fieldwork was over (Beebe, 2014).

Rapid Ethnographies

As mentioned in Chapter 1, there is variability in the use and definition of rapid ethnographies. I have discussed our typology of rapid ethnographies elsewhere (Vindrola-Padros, 2020; Vindrola-Padros and Vindrola-Padros, 2018), so for the purpose of this book, I have focused on highlighting the key features of four types of rapid ethnographies:

- ***Rapid ethnography:*** These approaches were carried out by lone researchers or by teams. They mainly included data collection methods commonly used in 'traditional' long-term ethnographic research (interviews, observations and documentary analysis), but involved short fieldwork periods. Rapid ethnographies have been used to study the implementation of patient portals in California (Ackerman et al., 2017), the use of clinical information systems by staff (Saleem et al., 2015), team dynamics in primary care practices (Chesluk and Holmboe, 2010), barriers to clubfoot treatment adherence in Uganda (McElroy et al., 2007), barriers to healthcare in Mozambique (Schwitters et al., 2015) and disparities in polio eradication (Hussain et al., 2015).
- ***Quick ethnography:*** Normally associated with the work of Handwerker (2001), quick ethnography was defined as 'a package that integrates conventional means of collecting cultural data [...], analysing cultural data (like grounded theory forms of text analysis and conventional statistics), and project management (like Gantt and PERT charts) with more novel forms of data collection (like successive pile sorts) and analysis (like the application

of multivariate statistical procedures to similarities among informants)' (Handwerker, 2001: 4). Handwerker (2001) defined ethnographic research as a mixed-methods approach, so many of his methodological recommendations involved the combination of qualitative and quantitative data. A recent study using quick ethnography was the use of human-centred design in cancer care (Mullaney et al., 2012).

- ***Focused ethnography:*** One way to reduce the length of time required for fieldwork has been by reducing the number of topics or areas under study and focusing the research questions. Focused ethnographies are 'selected, specified, that is, focused aspects of a field' (Knoblauch, 2005: 9). They are characterised by short-term field visits, a researcher with insider or background knowledge of the topic or cultural group and intensive methods of data collection and recording (i.e. video or audio-taping) (Wall, 2015). Focused ethnographies have been used to explore processes of teaching and learning in conflict zones (Skårås, 2018), describe the experiences of illness of homeless youths (Ensign and Bell, 2004), health-related perceptions and experiences of immigrant Latino adolescents (Garcia and Saewyc, 2007) and internationally educated nurses' transitioning experiences on relocation to Canada (Higginbottom, 2011). Focused ethnographies can be carried out by lone researchers, but recent studies have also explored team-based focused ethnography designs (for example, see Bikker et al., 2017).
- ***Short-term ethnography:*** This approach depended on the search for opportunities to use high-intensity fieldwork to collect in-depth and larger volumes of data over compressed timeframes (Pink and Morgan, 2013). Fieldwork was more targeted and visual methods (particularly video) were seen as helpful in facilitating data collection during these stages of high-intensity work (Pink and Morgan, 2013). Short-term ethnographies have a strong connection to theoretical invigoration (Pink and Morgan, 2013; Vindrola-Padros, 2020).

Rapid Evaluations

Rapid evaluations are different to other rapid qualitative approaches in the sense that they are designed with the specific purpose of assessing the impact or documenting the implementation of specific interventions, services or programmes (Vindrola-Padros et al., 2020). Even though some of these might have more exploratory designs, their ultimate aim is to explore the underlying assumptions guiding a service or intervention, the changes that need to take place, the mechanisms through which these might be achieved and the impact (or perceived impact) of these changes. Rapid evaluations might include an analysis of:

- Programme theories or logic models guiding the intervention design and its intended outcomes and their changes through time
- The processes used to implement interventions or services and the factors acting as barriers and facilitators
- The perceived impact of the implementation of the intervention or service on the intended outcomes

- The unintended consequences of implementing the intervention or service
- The experiences of those delivering or receiving the intervention or service
- The interaction of the intervention or service with components of the larger system to capture potential strategies for scale-up and long-term sustainability

Our recent review on the use of rapid evaluations in health services research found three frequently used types of evaluation designs: rapid evaluation methods (REMs), rapid feedback evaluation (RFE) and rapid cycle evaluation (RCE) (Vindrola-Padros et al., 2021). In addition to these, we have also found studies described as real-time evaluations (RTEs) and using rapid assessment methods (RAMs). Table 2.5 describes the different approaches and identifies some key literature.

Table 2.5 Common rapid evaluation designs

Evaluation design	Description	Key literature
Rapid evaluation methods (REMs)	Set of observation and survey-based diagnostic activities, which provide a basis for identifying operational problems and taking action	Anker et al. (1993); Aspray et al. (2006); Chowdhury and Moni (2004); Felisberto et al. (2008); Grant et al. (2011); Munday et al. (2018); Pearson (1989)
Rapid feedback evaluation (RFE)	Data are continually collected, analysed and used to inform action within a short time period. Aims at providing programme managers with focused, timely evaluation conclusions	Bjornson-Benson et al. (1993); Hargreaves (2014); McNall et al. (2004); Zakocs et al. (2015)
Rapid cycle evaluation (RCE)	Provides timely feedback to funding organisations and programme staff and care providers. Offers support for continuous quality improvement and allows observations of changes over time	Keith et al. (2017); McNall and Foster-Fishman (2007); Schneeweiss et al. (2015); Shrank (2013); Skillman et al. (2019)
Rapid assessment methods (RAM)	Enable gathering of valid and reliable research data within a rapid timeframe, and at relatively low cost	Pearson and Kessler (1992); Stimson et al. (1997); Vincent et al. (2000)
Real-time evaluation (RTE)	Based on sharing observations and recommendations on an ongoing basis with field staff so as to allow operational problems to be quickly corrected and potential problems to be avoided	Jamal and Crisp (2002); McNall and Foster-Fishman (2007); Sandison (2003); UNHCR (2002)

Source: Vindrola-Padros (2020).

Other Approaches and Hybrids

Even though many of the approaches discussed earlier are related and there has been a lot of cross-fertilisation between approaches, there are some rapid qualitative research methodologies that could be classified as more hybrid forms of rapid research. These include:

- ***Sondeo:*** A system approach to rapid research with the aim of obtaining a holistic understanding of a local situation. This approach was proposed by Hildebrand in the late 1970s and it has been mainly associated with farming systems research (Hildebrand, 1979).
- ***Micro-ethnography or mini-ethnography:*** These terms were used to describe ethnographies that were focused, with relatively small sample sizes or short amount of fieldwork (Storesund and McMurray, 2009). Fieldwork was guided by specific pre-formulated questions (Leininger, 1985; Werner and Schoepfle, 1987). These terms have also been used to describe the study of a single social situation (Spradley, 1980).
- ***Focused rapid ethnographic evaluation (FREE):*** This is a modification of the focused ethnography approach and it involved the extensive use of fieldnotes instead of digital recordings (Patmon et al., 2016). According to the designers of the approach, FREE was useful for analysing human–computer interactions and the assessment of emerging technologies in the workplace (Patmon et al., 2016).
- ***Short-term focused video ethnographic case study:*** This approach combined video footage, observational fieldnotes and postnatal video-cued interviews to provide in-depth analysis of one case study or situation. Harte et al. (2016) have used it to explore the hospital design factors influencing childbirth supporters' experiences.
- ***Rapid Assessment Procedure Informed Clinical Ethnography (RAPICE):*** The RAPICE has been recently developed in the field of clinical trials (Palinkas and Zatzick, 2019) to collect and use qualitative data to understand trial implementation processes and address barriers to recruitment and other issues. It combined some of the characteristics of RAPs outlined earlier (i.e. multidisciplinary research teams, use of several data collection methods, iterative collection and analysis and short study timeframes) with intensive participant observation normally used in clinical ethnography (Zatzick et al., 2011). Study findings were shared regularly with the trial team to inform changes in trial delivery (Palinkas and Zatzick, 2019).

A Continuum of Rapid Qualitative Research

A question that I often receive when I deliver courses on rapid qualitative research is 'out of all of the approaches you presented, which is the best one?' My answer is normally that it depends on the research questions guiding the study, the overall aim of the study (i.e. diagnosis, evaluation), the resources (including time) available for the study and the ways in which findings will be used. I also indicate that the distinctions between many of these approaches are not clear, as several are related or have suffered transformations over time. Instead of a black and white distinction (i.e. you can only use PRA for participatory research), I encourage colleagues to think about rapid qualitative research approaches on a continuum, where each approach might occupy different positions depending on the variable of interest, and where you might borrow features from multiple approaches to satisfy your study needs. Table 2.6 presents the approaches discussed in the chapter and a summary of their main characteristics.

Table 2.6 A summary of rapid qualitative research approaches and their main features

Name	Definition	Main uses	Data collection/ analysis structure	Lone researcher or team-based	Characteristics of the team	Sharing of findings	Key literature
Rapid rural appraisal (RRA)	'A strategy for appraising a particular situation in the most cost-effective manner possible with appropriate levels of timeliness, accuracy and relevance' (Heywood, 1990: 46)	Diagnostic or rapid assessment	A mixture of qualitative research methods	Team-based	Use of research teams with a high level of expertise and research skills with some input from local community members	Shared on an ongoing basis	Chambers (1981); Heywood (1990); Manderson and Aaby (1992a)
Participatory rural appraisal (PRA)	'A family of approaches and methods to enable rural people to share, enhance and analyse their knowledge of life and conditions, to plan and to act' (Chambers, 1994: 953)	Diagnostic or rapid assessment	Chambers has listed over 29 methods that can be used	Team-based	Community involvement in the gathering and analysis of data	Shared on an ongoing basis and community members can be involved in the analysis and interpretation of data	Chambers (1994); Rifkin (1992)

(Continued)

Table 2.6 (Continued)

Name	Definition	Main uses	Data collection/ analysis structure	Lone researcher or team-based	Characteristics of the team	Sharing of findings	Key literature
Rapid ethnographic assessment (REA)	A phenomenological method for rapid acquisition of data that are rich in life experiences of the subject population (Bentley et al., 1988)	Originally developed to provide quick assessments on local conditions to inform the design and implementation of interventions	Uses structured tools such as field guides	Team-based	Teams of four to eight people	Normally shared once the study is complete	Bentley et al. (1988); Sangaramoorthy and Kroeger (2020)
Rapid assessment procedure (RAP)	A way of gathering, analysing and interpreting high-quality ethnographic data expeditiously so that action can be taken as quickly as possible	Limited or focused scope of information to assist in problem solving	Uses a mix of qualitative and quantitative methods Uses structured tools such as field manuals	Team-based	More than one researcher is involved in data collection and analysis Involvement of decision makers at different levels: produce change and ensure credibility	Normally shared once the study is complete	Manderson and Aaby (1992a); Scrimshaw and Hurtado (1987)

Name	Definition	Main uses	Data collection/ analysis structure	Lone researcher or team-based	Characteristics of the team	Sharing of findings	Key literature
Rapid assessment, response and evaluation (RARE)	Systematic ethnographic data collection and analysis techniques complemented by survey information and direct observation studies	It is designed to be highly targeted and produces practical adaptable intervention recommendations that are correct for local conditions	Combine focus groups, key informant interviews, observations, mapping and rapid 'street intercept' assessment interviews. RARE manuals have been developed	Team-based	Team is led by a researcher with expertise in ethnography and includes community members as researchers	Findings are shared regularly with key stakeholders throughout the project	Brown et al. (2008); Needle et al. (2003)
Rapid qualitative inquiry (RQI) and rapid appraisals	'Intensive, team-based qualitative inquiry with a) a focus on the insider's or emic perspective, b) using multiple sources and triangulation, and c) using iterative data analysis and additional data collection to quickly develop a preliminary understanding of a situation' (Beebe, 2014, p. 6)	Diagnostic or rapid assessment	Data collection and analysis using triangulation Iterative process (several cycles of collection and analysis)	Team-based	Diversity (team members who are looking for different things) Multiple disciplines Insiders/outsiders Minimum of two team members and up to five members	Data collection and analysis are carried out iteratively so emerging findings can be shared on an ongoing basis	Beebe (1995, 2001, 2014)

(Continued)

Table 2.6 (Continued)

Name	Definition	Main uses	Data collection/ analysis structure	Lone researcher or team-based	Characteristics of the team	Sharing of findings	Key literature
Rapid ethnographies	Develop a reasonable understanding, in a compressed period of time, of the people and contexts being studied. Gather rich data without extended period of time in the field (Handwerker, 2001)	Exploratory, diagnostic, in-depth analysis, and some recent examples of evaluation	Based on the combination of different methods for data collection and triangulation. Can use structured tools but tends to rely more on unstructured approaches	Can use lone researchers or teams of researchers	Varies depending on the study, but some authors have argued in favour of having at least one social scientist with experience in ethnographic research	Findings can be shared after the study is complete or can be shared on an ongoing basis	Handwerker (2001); Knoblauch (2005); Pink and Morgan (2013); Vindrola-Padros (2020); Wall (2015)
Rapid evaluations	'Evaluation model that is focused on a particular issue, problem or information need, where evaluative information is needed in a short timeframe' (McNall et al., 2004: 288)	Evaluation of programmes, interventions or services	Combination of different methods for data collection and triangulation (can be mixed-methods) Data collection and analysis carried out in parallel to share emerging findings	Generally team-based	Different methodological expertise and can include stakeholders as members of the team	Rapid cycle evaluation (RCE) and rapid feedback evaluation (RFE) rely on the use of feedback loops to share emerging findings on a regular basis	Keith et al. (2017); McNall and Foster-Fishman (2007); Schneeweiss et al. (2015); Shrank (2013); Skillman et al. (2019)

When considering rapid qualitative research along a participatory continuum, you would normally assume that approaches such as PRA and RARE would be on the high end of the spectrum as the active participation of community members/people where the research will take place is a core defining feature of these approaches. Other approaches such as REA, RAP and rapid evaluations might encourage a relatively high level of participation. Rapid ethnographies, in the form of short-term ethnography, focused ethnography and quick ethnography, could also be designed as participatory studies, but the examples of published rapid ethnographies point to research designs where the lone researcher or the research team tend to be the main people designing and implementing the studies.

A similar picture emerges when we look at rapid qualitative research on a team-based continuum. Rapid ethnographies might tend to use a lone researcher approach, with the exception of team-based ethnographies. Rapid appraisals, RAP and the RARE model would normally exhibit a high degree of team-based research as data collection and analysis through teams of researchers is a defining feature of these approaches to reduce the amount of time required for field research and add different perspectives to the process of interpretation.

When examining these approaches on a structured continuum we allude to use of structured forms of data collection and analysis. This could be the use of field manuals or guides, observation guides or checklists or codebooks during analysis. Rapid ethnographies tend to be more unstructured in their design, while structured forms of data collection are frequently used in REA, RAP and RARE. One reason for this could be that these three approaches tend to use teams to collect data, so structured forms of data collection are used as a way to maintain consistency across members of the field research team (see Chapter 4 for an in-depth discussion of these structured forms). Going back to the question of the best rapid qualitative research approach, I also tell colleagues that I base these classifications on the way these approaches have *mainly* been used so far, there are always exceptions to the rule and there is always potential to use them differently. How else would we engage in methodological innovation?

Chapter Summary

- Rapid qualitative research encompasses a wide range of research approaches developed as early as the 1970s.
- Many of these approaches have cross-fertilised and changed over time. As a consequence, many rapid qualitative research approaches share common features such as short study duration, team-based research (and the development of tools to ensure consistency across researchers), iterative designs (where data collection and analysis are carried out in parallel) and the sharing of findings as the study is ongoing with relevant stakeholders.

- Some approaches such as PRA and the RARE model have a high degree of participation from the communities/areas where the study takes place.
- RAP, REA and the RARE model tend to use more structured tools to collect and analyse data.
- Rapid ethnographies are often carried out by lone researchers (with the exception of team-based ethnographies).
- RAP, the RARE model and rapid appraisals depend heavily on the use of teams for data collection and analysis.
- Rapid evaluations tend to focus on the assessment of specific interventions or services and experiment with different ways of delivering findings at regular intervals through feedback loops or cycles.

Discussion Questions

1. Can you identify any trends in the ways in which we use rapid qualitative research from the 1970s until now?
2. Are there any gaps in the ways in which we are applying these approaches? If so, how could these gaps be addressed?
3. Can you think of a continuum of rapid qualitative research not discussed in the chapter?

Exercise 2

What Is the Most Suitable Rapid Research Approach for My Study?

In this chapter, I have discussed different approaches used in rapid qualitative research, their interrelationships and how they have changed through time.

Option A

Think about your own study and select two rapid qualitative research approaches discussed in the chapter. Make a brief outline of your study design considering what it would look like depending on:

- The degree to which your study depends on the active participation of communities/organisations or other stakeholders under study
- The use of a lone researcher versus team-based approach
- The use of structured versus unstructured approaches for data collection and analysis

How do these decisions vary by approach? Which approach is more suitable for your study? Write a few lines justifying your decision.

Option B

Read the description of the study below and select **two** rapid qualitative research approaches discussed in the chapter that could be used to answer the research questions. Make a brief outline of the study design considering what it would look like depending on:

- The degree to which the study depends on the active participation of communities/organisations or other stakeholders under study
- The use of a lone researcher versus team-based approach
- The use of structured versus unstructured approaches to data collection and analysis

How do these decisions vary by approach? Which of the two approaches is more suitable for the study? Write a few lines justifying your decision.

The purpose of the study is to explore the main components of diabetes care for care-home residents and identify any barriers to care for this vulnerable population. Three questions will guide the study:*

1. What are residents' experiences of care?
2. What is the level of knowledge and attitudes of staff delivering diabetes care to this population?
3. What are the recommendations that can be made to the care home for improving care?

**Modified from the study published by Aspray et al. (2006).*

3

DESIGNING RAPID QUALITATIVE STUDIES

One of the lessons I have learnt is that rapid research normally requires more time and effort during the design phase than during data collection and analysis. I think that one of the reasons for this is that time for data collection is often considered a precious resource, so the study needs to be planned carefully to make sure time is used appropriately. In this chapter, I will describe some of the strategies we have used to make sure we follow an informed study design process, rapidly collect available evidence, engage with relevant stakeholders, anticipate challenges and develop strategies to mitigate risks.

Preparatory Work

Reviews of Existing Evidence

Topics for rapid qualitative studies might arise from our interest or we might be approached to carry out studies on topics where evidence is required to inform decision-making processes. Regardless of how a topic for a study has emerged, the first step we normally take is to search for literature (published or grey literature) on the topic. Our review of available evidence takes different forms and it is helpful to think of the different approaches we have used by placing them on a structured/unstructured spectrum. All of the searching we do is systematic (in the sense that it has been carried out in a transparent way so it can be replicated), but the way in which we approach reviewing, the synthesis and dissemination of findings will vary in terms of structure. In Table 3.1, I have included the main types of reviews and organised them across this spectrum.

Table 3.1 Evidence review approaches used in rapid qualitative research

Spectrum	Review Approach	Main Characteristics
Unstructured	Evidence mapping exercise	Evidence maps have been defined as 'a systematic search of a broad field to identify gaps in knowledge and/or future research needs that presents results in a user-friendly format, often a visual figure or graph, or a searchable database' (Miake-Lye et al., 2016: 18). The main differences between evidence mapping and other exploratory searching strategies, such as scoping reviews, lies in the robustness of their search strategy and the production of a visual or searchable database or diagram that is more 'user friendly' (Miake-Lye et al. 2016).
	Scoping review	A scoping review has been defined as 'a form of knowledge synthesis that addresses an exploratory research question aimed at mapping key concepts, types of evidence, and gaps in research related to a defined area or field by systematically searching, selecting, and synthesising existing knowledge' (Colquhoun et al., 2014: 1291). We normally follow the approaches established by Arksey and O'Malley (2005) and/or Levac et al. (2010). We tend to carry out scoping reviews when we want to map key concepts or types of evidence. We might also opt for a scoping review design if working in a very broad field where we might need to run multiple phases of searching to make sure we have identified as much of the available evidence as possible (see for instance Wood et al., 2018). We follow the PRISMA ScR statement (Tricco et al., 2018).
	Rapid systematic review	Rapid reviews have been defined as 'a type of knowledge synthesis in which components of the systematic review process are simplified or omitted to produce information in a short period of time' (Khangura et al., 2012: 8). For this type of review, we normally follow the rapid review method proposed by Tricco et al. (2017) for rapid evidence synthesis. The rapid review method follows a systematic review approach, but proposes adaptations to some of the steps to reduce the amount of time required to carry out the review (i.e. the use of large teams to review abstracts and full texts, and extract data; in lieu of dual screening and selection, a percentage of excluded articles is reviewed by a second reviewer, and software is used for data extraction and synthesis, as appropriate).

Spectrum	Review Approach	Main Characteristics
Structured	Systematic review	These tend to be longer reviews but we have still managed to carry out systematic reviews in rapid qualitative studies. We use the Preferred Reporting Items for Systematic Reviews and Meta-Analysis (PRISMA) statement (Moher et al., 2009) to guide the reporting of the methods and findings. If the review focuses on a health-related topic we register the review protocol with PROSPERO.

Scoping Phase

The scoping phase is a short stage prior to study design where we collect evidence from different sources and use this to inform the study design. This phase can be guided by a series of exploratory questions such as:

1. What is the main purpose of the study? What is it trying to inform?
2. Who are the main stakeholders?
3. What are the main components/factors shaping the area or situation under study?
4. What is the existing evidence in relation to this topic or area? What are the theoretical frameworks that have been used in previous studies?
5. Are there any overlapping or competing studies?
6. When do key decisions need to be made? Who will be involved in these decisions?
7. How will the research findings be used to inform these decisions? Are there any preferences in relation to the format or mechanism for sharing these findings?

These questions can be answered through a review of the literature using the approaches outlined earlier, but will tend to involve other types of data collection such as conversations with relevant stakeholders and, sometimes, other research teams, informal observations during key meetings, review of meeting minutes, review of theoretical frameworks, attending key events or carrying out tours of areas that will be studied later, and other activities where we could get a sense of the topic or area under study. We have developed a basic template for scoping phases composed of the following activities:

1. Meetings or informal telephone conversations with key stakeholders (five to seven people or more depending on the perspectives/views that need to be included) to obtain information on the context, current state of the programme/service or area under study and key activities (to answer the questions listed earlier)
2. Observations during relevant meetings and/or a tour of the area where the study will take place
3. Review of relevant documents (produced locally)
4. Informal conversations with research teams working on similar topics/areas
5. Rapid review of theoretical frameworks used previously in studies on the same topic/area

We tend to adapt this structure for each study as we might need to add events or data sources, but this structure allows us to capture a general idea of perceptions of the topic, practices and some retrospective data. Scoping phases vary in duration and this depends on the aims of the scoping but also the amount of time available for the complete study. We have carried out scoping phases in as little as five days and as long as six weeks. I have included an example of a scoping timeline in Table 3.2.

Table 3.2 Example of a scoping phase timeline

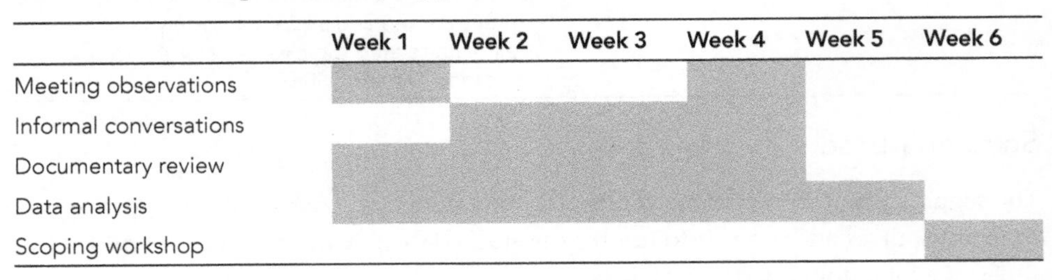

	Week 1	Week 2	Week 3	Week 4	Week 5	Week 6
Meeting observations	■			■		
Informal conversations		■	■	■		
Documentary review	■	■	■	■		
Data analysis	■	■	■	■	■	
Scoping workshop						■

As the name implies, the aim of the scoping phase is to delineate the scope of the study. This can be done entirely by the research team or in collaboration with others. We rarely define the scope of a study in isolation, so the scoping stage for us will often involve one or multiple meetings or workshops with stakeholders to discuss the scoping phase aims and findings. These findings are shared in the form of short reports, tables or slides. The meetings with stakeholders are used to discuss the findings and make joint decisions in relation to the research questions that will guide the rapid qualitative study, the study design and the key time points when the findings will be needed to inform decisions. The type of findings shared will vary by study but we have used scoping phases to share findings on:

1. The draft programme theory or model guiding the design of an intervention or programme
2. Areas or topics that stakeholders agree should be studied and areas of disagreement
3. The main problems outlined by key stakeholders and potential areas for improvement
4. Differences in perceptions/experiences across potential participant groups
5. Available data sources and potential issues accessing data in the rapid qualitative study
6. Areas or topics that might already be evaluated or studied by other teams
7. Theoretical frameworks that can be used to guide or frame the study
8. Preferences for dissemination, including a draft dissemination plan with a timeline

We normally present these findings, allow time for discussion and might use the time during scoping meetings or workshops with stakeholders to facilitate decision-making in relation to the study design through some form of participatory technique. The techniques we have used in the past have included:

- ***Ranking exercises:*** This exercise is used to facilitate the identification of research priorities so these priorities can be considered by the research team when designing the study protocol. It involves the following steps:
  - We present attendees with a potential list of areas that could be included in the study. We indicate that we cannot include everything due to limited time and resources.

- Participants are asked to think through the options and choose their favourite ones.
- We ask who would like to act as a sponsor for each area and 'pitch' the idea to the rest of the group. The 'pitch' entails identifying the main reasons why the area should be included in the study, the benefits it will create for stakeholders and reasons why other areas are not as important. This is done for all of the areas attributed some degree of importance by attendees (some might be eliminated even before the pitches begin).
- The list is put up on a large poster or flipchart paper. Attendees are given small circular stickers and asked to stick them next to the areas they think should be prioritised. Attendees receive the number of stickers the research team think is appropriate for the number of areas they would like to include. In other words, if researchers think the top three areas can be included in the study, then attendees receive three stickers.
- Attendees analyse the placement of stickers and come to an agreement on the areas that need to be prioritised.

- ***Important/urgent piles:*** This exercise can be used in combination with the ranking exercise described earlier to further classify priority areas as important or urgent, or it can be used as a standalone exercise. The purpose of this exercise is to get a sense of how areas might need to be included in the study to make sure findings are shared at a time when they can be used to inform key decisions. It can also help the research team to decide how much time and effort should be dedicated to study each area. It involves the following steps:
  - The research team develops cards with the key areas that could be included in the study or these areas are identified at the workshop by attendees themselves through a free listing exercise (see Chapter 4). If this is a large group, several copies of the cards need to be developed so attendees can work in smaller groups.
  - When looking through the cards, attendees need to ask themselves the following question: is this something we need to know now or can we know about this later? If the answer is now, then the area needs to be placed in the 'urgent pile'. Attendees might also want to ask themselves, do I think this is important because it needs to be done now, or is this important beyond this sense of urgency? If the answer is the latter, then the area can be placed in the 'important pile'.
  - After the attendees have gone through all of the cards and organised them into piles (attendees might be allowed to create a third 'maybe' or 'unsure' pile as well), the facilitators will review all piles and develop a table that needs to be seen by everyone (either projected on a screen or written on a flipchart). The table will need to include the following columns: areas we all agree are urgent, areas we all agree are important, areas of disagreement and areas where we are unsure.
  - The facilitators can then moderate a discussion in relation to these areas until agreement is reached. The research team will then need to make a decision, with the agreement of the attendees, in relation to how to integrate these urgent/important categories in the study. This will depend on the time and resources available for the study, but some ways in which we have done this in the past include:
    - Only include important areas and leave urgent areas out of the study. We did this in studies where we did not have many resources for the study.

    - Include urgent and important areas and design the study so findings relevant for the urgent areas can be delivered first.
    - Include urgent and important areas, but automatically exclude those where there was disagreement or where attendees grouped them in the 'unsure' pile.
    - Only include urgent areas and use these study findings to design a longer study that can cover the important areas.
- ***How would we use the findings?:*** The purpose of this exercise is to get attendees to prioritise areas for research that will generate the findings that they need at that time. It includes the following steps:
    - The research team develops cards with the key areas that could be included in the study or these areas are identified at the workshop by attendees themselves through a free listing exercise (see Chapter 4). If this is a large group, several copies of the cards need to be developed so attendees can work in smaller groups. Attendees are given stacks of blank cards and markers.
    - Attendees are asked to look at the cards and ask themselves, if the team study this area, what type of findings would we get? They are asked to write this down and place it next to the area card. They are requested to ask themselves, how will we use these findings? They are asked to write their answer down in a separate card and place it next to the 'types of findings card'. Attendees would then have a row in front of them, composed of three columns created with an area card, a type of findings card and 'a how we will use the findings card'.
    - The research team will take the 'how we will use the findings' card and make sure to add details of the area these belong to on the back. The team will combine all 'how we will use the findings' cards from all sub-groups. They will present these to the team and ask them to rank the 'how we will use the findings' cards based on the priorities of the group. A general question about importance can be asked to facilitate the ranking process or this exercise can be combined with the important/urgent piles exercise described earlier.
    - After the top 'how we will use the findings' cards are identified, the team will turn them over to show the areas they are related to. The team will then facilitate an open discussion in relation to these to see if attendees agree that they are areas that need to be included in the study. It might be that several of the 'how we will use them' cards relate to the same area and this is fine as it confirms the importance of this area. It could also be that areas considered important by some attendees do not appear at this stage. This open discussion can be used to present these additional areas and reach an agreement as a group. As long as attendees have been able to think through the types of findings generated for each area and how they will use them, this exercise will have reached its ultimate goal.

In addition to the identification of these areas of research, the final outcome of the scoping is a general agreement in relation to the research questions, study design and dissemination plan that we will translate into a written proposal and circulate to all stakeholders for final sign-off. The process of developing these proposals entails making the decisions in relation to study design and dissemination outlined in the following sections.

Focusing the Research Questions

Even though there is variability across rapid qualitative research approaches, most of these approaches rely on the use of focused research questions to make sure they can be answered within limited timeframes for data collection and analysis. The scoping phase described earlier can help focus the questions as the research team would have a better idea of the priorities of the study, areas that have already been covered/studied and ways in which findings will be used. Authors such as Knoblauch (2005) and Wall (2015), through their work on focused ethnographies, have highlighted a series of conditions for focusing research questions. It is easier to focus questions when the research team has some previous knowledge or experience with the topic or area under study. Focused research questions tend to explore 'situations, interactions and activities' (Knoblauch, 2005) rather than broader fields of inquiry such as particular settings, groups, organisations or communities. Furthermore, rapid qualitative research will aim to explore specific aspects of these situations, interactions and activities, delineated by time (i.e. capturing a 'snapshot' of activity), determined by the theoretical framework used in the study and its creation of a 'particular lens' to collect and analyse data, or influenced by the type of findings that will be useful for informing decisions. For example, instead of framing a study to explore nursing practice in acute care hospitals, a rapid qualitative study might focus on the delivery of one-to-one care to patients at risk of falls hospitalised in 'care of the elderly' wards within acute care hospitals.

Choosing the Rapid Approach

As discussed in Chapter 2, the field of rapid qualitative research is diverse and includes a wide range of approaches. The selection of approaches will ultimately depend on the research questions, but can also vary in relation to the duration of the study, available resources, team composition, degree of flexibility and general preferences and experience of the researchers. In order to facilitate the selection of an approach, I have developed the decision tool included in Table 3.3. The tool includes the questions we ask ourselves before selecting an approach and the potential choices based on the answers to these questions. It is related to the discussion on the continuum in rapid qualitative research presented in Chapter 2.

In addition to these questions, researchers will also need to consider the research questions, resources available for the study and the total duration of the study. It is important to consider that these are only suggestions made based on the most common uses of

Table 3.3 Decision tool for the selection of rapid qualitative research approaches

RREAL RAPID QUALITATIVE RESEARCH DECISION TOOL

This tool is a flexible guide based on the frequent application of these approaches. Some of these approaches can be used across all of the categories identified in the tool.

Questions to guide study design	Types of rapid qualitative research approaches		
AIM	**Diagnostic purposes:** rapid appraisal, RRA	**Exploration or to seek understanding:** rapid ethnography, RQI	**Evaluation:** rapid evaluations, RAP
How participatory?	**High degree of participation:** PRA, RARE	**Medium degree of participation:** Rapid appraisal, RQI	**Low degree of participation:** rapid ethnography, rapid evaluations
How structured?	**Structured:** RAP, REA	**Somewhat structured:** rapid evaluations, rapid appraisals, RQI, RRA, PRA	**Unstructured:** rapid ethnographies
Team or lone researcher?	**Team-based:** rapid appraisals, RQI, RARE, RAP, team-based rapid ethnographies		**Lone researcher:** rapid ethnographies and some types of rapid evaluations
When are findings needed? (one time-point or regular feedback?)	**Regular feedback:** rapid feedback or rapid cycle evaluations, rapid appraisals, RAP, RARE, rapid ethnographies		**One-time feedback:** REM, rapid ethnographies

RAP: Rapid Assessment Procedure

RARE: Rapid Assessment Response and Evaluation

RQI: Rapid Qualitative Inquiry

REA: Rapid Ethnographic Assessment

RRA: Rapid Rural Appraisal

PRA: Participatory Rural Appraisal

Visual abstract design: Franco Marquez

these approaches as reported in the literature. For instance, I propose the use of rapid ethnographies in the case of lone researcher teams, but some researchers might also need to carry out rapid evaluations as lone researchers. Furthermore, in practice, the boundaries between approaches are permeable and arbitrary and we often combine features and tools from different research approaches in the same study.

Selecting and Combining the Methods

Chapters 4 and 5 are dedicated to the exploration of the most common methods used for data collection and analysis and how these have been adapted for rapid qualitative designs. In this section, I only allude to general aspects of study design that might be relevant for rapid qualitative studies regardless of the methods used for data collection and analysis.

Triangulation

As mentioned in Chapter 2, most rapid qualitative research approaches tend to be multi-layered in their designs, as they might combine multiple researchers, data sources and interpretive lenses. Beebe (2001: 20) has argued that rapid assessment processes can combine five types of triangulation:

- Data triangulation based on the use of different data sources
- Investigator triangulation where multiple researchers are used to collect and analyse data
- Theory triangulation to bring together multiple perspectives to interpret the same data
- Methodological triangulation by using multiple methods
- Interdisciplinary triangulation where researchers from different disciplines collect and analyse data from multiple perspectives, generating additional layers of meaning (see also Denzin & Lincoln, 1995)

Triangulation should not be confused with the accumulation of data as the goal of triangulation is not to increase the volume of data. On the contrary, it seeks to explore how different sources of data intertwine to generate insight, confirm assumptions or contradict each other. Furthermore, different theoretical perspectives and the points of view of researchers from different disciplines will allow teams to identify multiple ways of 'cutting the data' or interpreting the findings.

Iterative Designs

One of the key defining features of rapid qualitative research is its iterative design (Beebe, 2001; McNall and Foster-Fishman, 2007). Iterative designs refer to the repetitive, circular and constantly changing process of research, where cycles are built into the study to transition from study design, data collection, analysis, reflection in relation to changes that might need to be made in the design and beginning the cycle all over again. In the case of rapid qualitative research, I have identified four layers of iteration (see Figure 3.1). The scoping phase shapes the first layer of iteration, where the researcher draws from available published and verbally communicated evidence to create initial drafts of the study design, discusses these with stakeholders and makes adaptations.

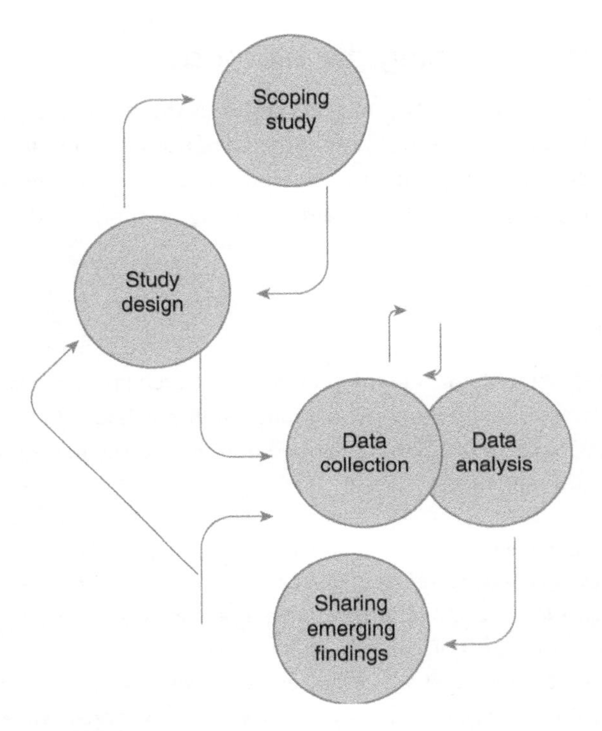

Figure 3.1 Layers of iteration in rapid qualitative research

A second layer is added once the study begins. Data are analysed as data collection is still ongoing, the analysis points to ways in which data collection needs to be changed or adapted. This could entail modifying the sampling framework to include new people to interview or events to observe or changing the questions included in interview topic guides. It can also mean more drastic changes such as adding additional sites to the study or removing methods for data collection that might not be working in practice.

Another layer of iteration has to do with the sharing of emerging findings. Many rapid qualitative research approaches carry out data collection and analysis in parallel to be able to share findings as the study is ongoing. This process of sharing might also entail obtaining feedback on the findings and the study progress from stakeholders. This feedback can then be used to make changes in the analysis of findings (focusing on areas that are of particular interest, seeking clarification in relation to specific topics or searching for completely new areas that were overlooked at the start of the study). The feedback from stakeholders might also lead to changes in the way in which the study is designed and data are collected.

The last layer might not be applicable to all studies and it will depend on the extent to which the researchers have designed the study to be responsive to changes in the local context. For those of us working in the healthcare sector, changes in the organisational and financial landscape mean that the context that we are studying can be changing drastically as the study is ongoing. This might mean, for instance, that the service or programme we were asked to study or evaluate might be interrupted or eliminated during our study, or healthcare organisations might be experiencing new pressures that lead to the changing of priorities and the shift in focus in the delivery of services (potentially requiring a similar shift in focus in our study). In a recent study, Bowen et al. (2019) found that senior leaders in healthcare organisations highlighted a mismatch between their evidence needs and health services research carried out in their organisations. The main reasons for this mismatch included the design of studies without considering the priorities and challenges of healthcare organisations and the inability to change the study at the same pace as the healthcare organisations adapted to their local context (Bowen et al., 2019). The mismatch led to the dissolution of provider–academic partnerships, the lack of use of research findings to inform decision-making and the prevalence of gaps in local knowledge (Bowen et al., 2019). I published a commentary in response to this article, arguing for the need to develop qualitative research that can be rapid, relevant and responsive (Vindrola-Padros, 2020). Responsiveness is closely related to this last stage of iteration, where the researchers are aware of changes happening at the organisational and system level and are prepared to adapt studies so these changes can be documented and incorporated in the study design.

Designing the Sampling Strategy

One of the challenges of carrying out rapid qualitative research identified in the literature is that shorter data collection periods might mean researchers rely on informants who are most accessible, losing the diversity of perspectives (i.e. in hard to reach populations) or conflicting points of view (Bentley et al., 1988; Harris et al., 1997; Manderson and Aaby, 1992a, 1992b; Pink and Morgan, 2013). Several approaches have been developed in the field of rapid research to mitigate these potential risks in sampling strategies. Rapid qualitative research uses sampling techniques that are common in qualitative research, where the aim of the sampling is to understand a wide range of perspectives or different dimensions of the local context (Sangaramoorthy and Kroeger, 2020). Therefore, two prevalent sampling approaches include purposive and snowball sampling. Purposive sampling focuses on the inclusion of participants, episodes, documents based on pre-established categories that are relevant to the research questions (Ritchie et al., 2004). By establishing relevant categories in advance, purposive sampling strategies seek to ensure there are no gaps in data collection.

In order to facilitate purposive sampling, researchers often create sampling frameworks, frames or briefs similar to the one included in Table 3.4. Tables such as this one make the research team consider the key people that will need to be included in the interviews, sampling, for instance, across professional groups, levels of seniority, sites and time points. Sampling frameworks can also help researchers address the challenges involved in sampling in rapid research outlined earlier, where, by following the framework, researchers would aim to meet the sampling targets, rather than only recruiting participants who are easier to reach or observing the events that are most accessible (leaving out key points of view or situations). Researchers might want to add more detail to their framework than I have presented in Table 3.4, making sure they include any variables in relation to, for instance, gender, amount of time working on the ward, specialty and so on.

Table 3.4 Example of a sampling framework for interviews

	Sites		
Hospital professional group	**A**	**B**	**C**
Junior nurses	3	3	3
Senior nurses	2	2	2
Junior doctors	3	3	3
Senior doctors	2	2	2
Ward managers	1	1	1
Domestic staff	2	2	2
Total	**13**	**13**	**13**

It is important to note that sampling frameworks are not set in stone and can be changed as the study is ongoing to add or remove categories of people, events or documentary evidence. Snowball sampling is sometimes combined with purposive sampling to inform these changes in the sampling framework. Snowball sampling consists of the recruitment of a few key participants to the study and asking them to recommend other relevant people who should be approached to take part in the study (Ritchie et al., 2004). The sample will then be expanded to include these participants and, as these new participants are asked to recommend additional people, the sample will continue to grow. When combined with purposive sampling, snowball sampling allows researchers to cross-check their initial sampling categories, confirming those that were initially included and adding any that were not originally identified by the research team. In the case of rapid qualitative research, snowball sampling is also helpful in the sense that sampling is taking place in parallel to data collection and analysis, allowing for three stages of research to happen simultaneously, thus saving time.

Sampling frameworks are not only useful for the sampling of individuals as presented in Table 3.4 but can also be used to sample study sites. Tables can be developed to organise the study sites based on the characteristics that might be of interest to the study. In

Table 3.5, I have included a sampling framework we developed to select hospitals that would be taking place in an evaluation of a national study that aimed to explore the impact of an intervention on how hospital data were used for local quality improvement. Our initial review of the data during the scoping phase pointed to potential variation in data collection and data use based on the geographic region where the hospital was situated, the type of hospital (teaching hospital or district general hospital) and sector (urban/rural). We also assumed that sites might present differences depending on how long they had been involved in the intervention and their degree of engagement. We considered all of these characteristics and selected sites that exhibited variation across all of them.

Table 3.5 Example of a sampling framework for study sites

	Long-term involvement		**Recent involvement**	
Criteria	**A**	**B**	**C**	**D**
Geographic location	North	South	Centre	North
Type	DGH	Teaching	DGH	Teaching
Size	Small	Large	Medium	Medium
Rural/urban	Rural	Urban	Urban	Urban
Engagement	Low	Medium	High	Low

DGH: District General Hospital.

In rapid qualitative research, we might not have enough time to collect in-depth data across all of the sites included in Table 3.5. One way we have addressed this is by developing smaller samples of sites (when compared to longer-term studies) to make sure we have enough time to visit all of them. Another option is to keep a large sample of sites, but carry out data collection during very short, but intensive, periods of fieldwork at each site. Halme et al. (2016), for instance, carried out data collection across four sites and were able to do this by arranging all data collection over a two- to four-week period.

Another way in which we sample sites to cover a broad range of contexts but keep data collection manageable is by developing a sample with different levels of depth. In a recent rapid evaluation of a national programme, we knew we needed to include sites across different geographical regions, in rural and urban settings and capturing a wide range of catchment areas and population sizes. Due to the short duration of the study (nine months) and the small size of the research team (two qualitative researchers), we knew we would not be able to carry out interviews, participant-observation and documentary analysis across all of them. We decided to carry out a site sampling strategy, including eight sites, four that would be labelled as 'in-depth sites' and four that would be labelled as 'high-level sites' (see Table 3.6). In the in-depth sites, we would apply all methods of data collection: face-to-face interviews, participant observation during team and department meetings, and documentary analysis of documents produced at hospital level. In the high-level sites, however, we would carry out the interviews remotely (via telephone) and we would not visit the sites to carry out observations of the meetings but would review the meeting notes or minutes instead. We would carry out the documentary analysis of other hospital documents in the same way as in the in-depth sites. We identified the limitations of this sampling strategy early on in the study design but decided that, despite not achieving the same degree of depth or understanding across all sites, it was preferable to at least have some level of insight across a variety of hospitals.

Table 3.6 Sampling study sites classified as in-depth and high-level sites

	In-depth sites				High-level sites			
Criteria	**A**	**B**	**C**	**D**	**E**	**F**	**G**	**H**
Geographic location	North	South	Centre	South	North	South	Centre	South
Type	DGH	Teaching	DGH	Teaching	Teaching	DGH	Teaching	DGH
Size	Small	Large	Medium	Large	Large	Small	Large	Small
Rural/urban	Rural	Urban	Urban	Urban	Urban	Rural	Urban	Rural

Most of the time, we refer to the use of sampling frameworks for individuals who will be recruited for interviews. However, I have often used sampling frameworks for observations and documents that will be included in documentary analysis. As mentioned earlier, the scoping phase will often include a tour of the area that will be studied. We use this tour and informal conversations with relevant stakeholders to map the situations, events or episodes that we might want to observe. We then develop a framework such as the one included in Table 3.7, where we organise these observation opportunities across sites, time points and researchers. Like the framework used for individuals, the sampling framework for observations is considered a working document by the team and will probably experience transformations as the study is ongoing.

Table 3.7 Example of a sampling framework for observations

Situation/Meeting	Number of sessions
Huddles	8
Multidisciplinary meetings	4
Department meetings	2
One-to-one interactions with patient	
- Bedside	5
- At discharge	5
Interactions with family members	5

A sampling framework for documents can be created in a similar way, with some early mapping of potential documents to review for the study during the scoping phase and a clear layout of what needs to be collected over time and/or across sites. This is particularly useful if the plan is to review different types of documents such as reports, meeting minutes, leaflets and letters. In a rapid appraisal of barriers to local quality improvement, we used the sampling framework in Table 3.8 to make sure we had collected all of the documents we needed before completing data collection.

Table 3.8 Example of sampling framework for documents used in a rapid appraisal

Document type	Site A	Site B	Site C
Trust quality improvement strategy	1	1	1
CQC report	Latest	Latest	Latest
Minutes from quality improvement committee meetings	All minutes for the past two years	All minutes for the past two years	All minutes for the past two years
Minutes from Board meetings	All minutes for the past two years	All minutes for the past two years	All minutes for the past two years
Examples of QI projects at ward or division level	3	3	3

Sampling frameworks can also be helpful when planning rapid qualitative studies that involve a series of short periods of data collection. These staggered fieldwork stages are normally used to capture changes over time. We use this design in rapid feedback and rapid cycle evaluations where we seek to track the implementation of an intervention or programme and understand if experiences and practices related to the intervention have changed over time. Table 3.9 includes a sampling framework we used to identify the time point when we would need to carry out data collection across 10 wards to make sure we captured all stages of the implementation of a hospital-wide intervention.

Table 3.9 Example of a sampling framework to stager wards based on time of intervention rollout

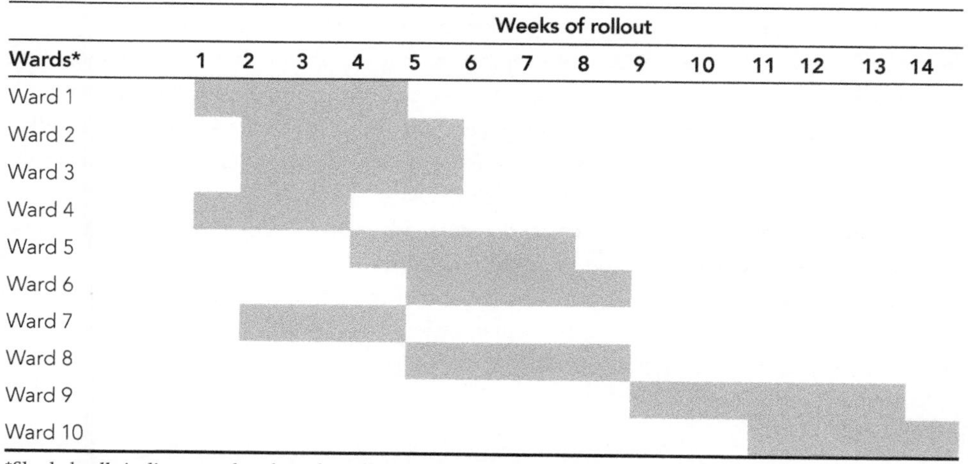

	Weeks of rollout													
Wards*	1	2	3	4	5	6	7	8	9	10	11	12	13	14
Ward 1	■	■	■	■										
Ward 2		■	■	■	■									
Ward 3		■	■	■	■									
Ward 4	■	■	■											
Ward 5				■	■	■	■							
Ward 6					■	■	■	■						
Ward 7		■	■	■										
Ward 8					■	■	■	■						
Ward 9									■	■	■	■	■	
Ward 10											■	■	■	■

*Shaded cells indicate weeks when the rollout would occur at each ward.

Developing the Dissemination Plans

I have dedicated an entire chapter to dissemination (Chapter 7) but the reason I bring up dissemination in this chapter is because it is a crucial aspect of the study design (although one that is often overlooked). In order for the study findings to be used to inform changes in practice and policy, dissemination needs to be discussed as early as the scoping phase. We often use the scoping phase to identify specific time points when findings might be needed to inform decisions. We make sure to plot these time points in our study timelines and, using the iterative study design described earlier, we make sure we are able to carry out data collection and analysis in parallel to share emerging findings by these deadlines.

Teams that have not included dissemination as part of the design will often think about sharing findings after data collection and analysis have ended, potentially presenting findings to stakeholders when it is too late. They might have also missed out on opportunities for obtaining feedback from stakeholders while the study was ongoing, feedback that could have led to the identification of other participants that needed to be included in the study or additional events that needed to be observed. In Chapter 7, I discuss the process of developing dissemination plans to avoid these missed opportunities.

Chapter Summary

- The design of rapid qualitative studies can be informed by preparatory work composed of a review of existing evidence and a scoping phase.
- The preparatory work helps with the identification of the theoretical framework/s that will guide the study and the focusing of the research questions so the study is targeted.
- A key aspect of the scoping phase is the engagement with key stakeholders to prioritise areas of research and the research questions, as well as agree the study design and dissemination plan.
- Rapid qualitative research approaches tend to combine the use of multiple methods for data collection and the use of triangulation for data analysis.
- Study designs in rapid qualitative research often involve different layers of iteration, where scoping phases inform the study design, data collection and analysis are carried out in parallel (also informing the study design) and the feedback obtained from stakeholders when sharing emerging findings can create an additional loop to prompt changes in the study design and data collection/analysis processes.
- Sampling frameworks for research participants, observations, documents and study sites can help researchers overcome sampling limitations in rapid qualitative studies.
- Different layers of iteration (at scoping stage, throughout data collection and when sharing emerging findings), need to be built into the study design.
- The development of a dissemination plan should be considered a stage in research design.

Discussion Questions

1. What are the main types of findings that can be generated during a scoping phase?
2. What are other ways in which patients and/or their families could be engaged in the research process (other than those mentioned in the book)?
3. What are some of the potential limitations or problems associated with the use of sampling frameworks in rapid qualitative research?

Exercise 3

Developing the Study Design

Option A

Think about your own study and develop an outline of the potential study design. Think about the following questions as you are developing the outline:

1. Do you need to carry out any scoping or other type of preparatory work to inform the design of your study?
2. Who are the key stakeholders you will need to engage during early stages of design?
3. What are the main research questions guiding your study? Are these focused enough for a rapid study?
4. You have already explored potential options in relation to rapid qualitative research approaches in Exercise 2. When using the decision tool (Table 3.3), what approach is more suitable for answering your research questions?
5. Develop a sketch of a potential dissemination plan.

Option B

Read the following case study and develop an outline of the potential study design. Think about the following questions as you are developing the outline:

1. Do you need to carry out any scoping or other type of preparatory work to inform the design of your study?
2. Who are the key stakeholders you will need to engage during the early stages of design?
3. What are the main research questions guiding your study? Are these focused enough for a rapid study?

4 You have already explored potential options in relation to rapid qualitative research approaches in Exercise 2. When using the decision tool (Table 3.3.), what approach is more suitable for answering your research questions?
5 Develop a sketch of a potential dissemination plan.

Case study: Programme to support parents of children with learning disabilities

A new programme aimed at supporting parents of children with learning disabilities is being rolled out across three neighbourhoods through their local community centres. Your team has been asked to develop a rapid qualitative study with the aim of documenting the process of implementation and capture lessons learnt that could be used to inform the rollout of the programme in other neighbourhoods.

Your team is composed of three full-time researchers. The study should not last more than six months and emerging findings need to be shared in two months to inform decisions that need to be made during the early implementation phase.

4

DATA COLLECTION IN RAPID QUALITATIVE RESEARCH

Rapid qualitative research approaches have included innovations in the development of methods for data collection over short periods of time. Many of these methods are frequently used in qualitative research but adaptations are proposed for rapid or intensive fieldwork stages. Many of these approaches also rely on the use of structured tools to speed up data collection and ensure consistency across field researchers when collecting data as a team. In this chapter, I provide an overview of the methods that have been used to collect data in rapid qualitative research. I focus on methods commonly used in qualitative research as well as those developed specifically for rapid research. I provide options for those carrying out research as lone researchers as well as those collecting data in teams.

How Do I Decide Which Methods to Use?

The best overview of data collection methods for rapid qualitative research, in my opinion, is the one published by Robert Chambers (1994) when comparing rapid rural appraisal (RRA) and participatory rural appraisal (PRA). Chambers argued that PRAs tended to avoid detailed handbooks or manuals of methods and relied more on the principle of 'use of your own best judgement at all time' (1994: 959). In this article, he sets out a sketch of potential methods with basic descriptions, encouraging readers to be creative in their application and combination. In Table 4.1, I have included the list of methods and Chambers' (1994) descriptions.

Table 4.1 List of methods for RRA and PRA proposed by Chambers (1994)

Method	Description/Examples
Secondary sources	Files, reports, maps, aerial photographs and satellite imagery
Key informant interviews	Enquiring those who are experts
Group interviews of various kinds	Can be casual or specific and structured to guide discussion on topics

(Continued)

Table 4.1 (Continued)

Method	Description/Examples
Do-it-yourself interviews	The researcher asks to be taught how to do something
They do it interviews	Community members carry out the data collection: observations, interviews and so on
Mapping and modelling	Community members make their own community maps or models of their land
Transect walks	Walking with community members to identify zones, problems and solutions
Timelines and trend analysis	Development of chronologies of events, recent changes
Oral histories and ethno biographies	Recording of local histories
Seasonal calendars	Recording of changes occurring by season or month to understand wider changes in the community
Daily time use analysis	Identifying the amount of time allocated for different activities and who is involved in these
Grouping and ranking methods	Grouping people or activities based on specific prompts. This approach can also be used to rank community members based on wealth, power, access and so on
Group discussions and brainstorming	Focus groups or group discussions led by external researcher or community members
Presentation analysis	Analysis of presentations delivered by community members on maps, diagrams or other materials from the community
Schedules for short and quick questionnaires	Quick surveys or questionnaires designed to collect targeted information from a large sample size
Protocols for observations	Structured tools to capture observations on specific issues and ensure all field researchers collect data in the same way

Our Rapid Interviewing Process

Interviews are one of the data collection methods most frequently used in qualitative research. In this book, I will not provide a general introduction to interviewing as this has already been done in various qualitative research methods books (Morse, 1994; Taylor et al., 2015). My aim in this section of the chapter is to describe the ways in which interviewing has been adapted to collect and analyse data rapidly. The process of interviewing can be carried out quickly by:

1. ***Limiting the scope of the interview to focus on few topics:*** These 'targeted interviews' are normally short in duration allowing researchers to cover more participants.
2. ***Using a large team to interview:*** More researchers cover more ground and the target sample size can be achieved quicker.
3. ***Carrying out data collection and analysis in parallel:*** If interviews are analysed almost in real time, the total amount of time for the study can be reduced.

These three strategies are not mutually exclusive and all three can be used in the same study. Limited or targeted interviews might not be possible for all studies and some research questions will need to be answered with in-depth and longer interviews. In these cases, the other two strategies can be used to save time. The use of a large team has benefits in terms of being able to interview a large group of research participants, but large teams of researchers are also difficult to manage and there might be difficulties ensuring consistency in the collected data. I will come back to this point later in the chapter when I discuss structured approaches and quality control and in Chapter 6 when I discuss the challenges of rapid qualitative research.

The third strategy, which is based on an iterative approach to data collection and analysis, is the one I have used with great frequency in rapid qualitative research. I have developed a process for rapid interviewing that has been used successfully in rapid appraisals, rapid ethnographies, rapid assessment procedures (RAPs) and rapid evaluations. This rapid approach to interviewing consists of the following steps:

1 ***Preparatory work:*** Reach agreement within the team in relation to the interview topic guide and the data the team expects to collect from the interviews.
2 ***During the interview:*** During the interview, each interviewer audio records the interview but also takes notes documenting the conversation. The notes are helpful for guiding the discussion, can act as a safety net in case the audio recorder fails, and allow the researcher to have a summary of the main findings at the end of the interview.
3 ***After the interview:*** The interviewer takes their notes and enters the main findings into a RAP sheet developed and agreed by the team. The original RAP sheet was used in RAPs to summarise all findings at the end of a study. In the case of our studies, RAP sheets are basically a simple table that includes the list of the main data we hope to obtain during data collection (see example in Table 4.2). After each interview, the interviewer enters a summary of the findings from their interview notes into the RAP sheet. This means that, at the end of each day of data collection, the team has a summary of the main findings from all of the interviews carried out to date. If data are being collected from different data sources (i.e. observations or documents), summaries of findings from these can be added to the same RAP sheet. The RAP sheet can then also act as a triangulation tool.
4 ***As interviews are ongoing:*** RAP sheets can be used as a way to cross-check data collection and ensure all researchers are collecting data in the same way. RAP sheets are flexible tools and we often modify them throughout the data collection stage, removing rows that no longer work or adding topics that we had not anticipated. RAP sheets can be used to identify gaps in data collection during fieldwork. New questions can be added to the interview topic guide or changes made to the sampling strategy to address these gaps before data collection is finished.
5 ***After data collection is complete:*** As all interviews are audio recorded, the team will have the choice of carrying out full or selected transcription during or after data collection. RAP sheets can also be used as a way to identify salient topics and then go back to transcripts to get a clearer idea of the details. I describe the process of analysis in Chapter 5.

RAP sheets can be designed in different ways, depending on the aims of the study. If the study requires a comparison of data across different team members, then the team might want to use one RAP sheet per researcher. Having one RAP sheet per researcher allows the team to quickly look across all sheets and get a sense of findings emerging across the entire sample. If the study aims to compare findings across different research sites or cases, then the team would probably want to use one RAP sheet per study site. All researchers collecting data on this site would add this information to the same RAP sheet. Even if data are collected from multiple sources, these would all be added to the RAP sheet of the specific case or study site. This way, the RAP sheet brings together the findings generated by multiple researchers and multiple data collection methods. At the end of the fieldwork, the tables of each site can be placed together side by side to facilitate cross-case comparisons.

If the aim of the study is to compare findings across populations, then it might be more appropriate to develop a RAP sheet per group included in the sample (i.e. for doctors, nurses, patients, etc.). The process would be the same as the one described for the site-based RAP sheets earlier. RAP sheets can also be used to view changes over time, where each RAP sheet can be developed at a particular stage in the study and compared at the end. For instance, if the study is a rapid evaluation interested in capturing changes before and after the implementation of an intervention, the team can develop a RAP sheet for before the implementation stage and for one after and then compare findings across them.

One of the benefits of using this rapid interviewing process is the rapid identification of findings so they can be shared with stakeholders almost on a real-time basis. The close contact to the emerging findings allows teams to identify gaps in the collected data and address these as fieldwork is ongoing. By using the RAP sheets as flexible tools (adaptable and subject to change), rigid frameworks are not imposed on the data and the team are open to new topics emerging from the interviews. The potential problems with this approach include inconsistencies in the recording of interview notes and the entry of information into the RAP sheets. The use of tools such as the RAP sheet might also require the training of field researchers before fieldwork begins. Even though RAP sheets are considered as flexible tools, there is a risk of imposing pre-established ideas on the data collection process and missing important details from the interviews.

Focus Groups

Focus groups are often used in rapid qualitative research to capture the views of a wide range of individuals within a short timeframe. Focus groups are normally used to generate data through the interaction and conversations between individuals in small groups (Finch et al., 2003).

Forming the Groups

Rapid qualitative research has used similar approaches to recruit participants for focus groups as longer-term research, but some studies have also explored the use of natural groups and informal focus groups. Natural groups have been defined as 'those conducted with individuals who have not been assembled for the purpose of the study at hand but exist for some other reason' (Coreil et al., 1989: S35). These can be produced by individuals who come together unexpectedly (i.e. people waiting in line outside of a bank) or can be existing groups where individuals regularly come together for a specific non-research related purpose (i.e. parents who join baby playgroups). In their rapid ethnographic assessment (REA) of barriers to health service use in Haiti, Coreil et al. (1989) interviewed four natural groups of mothers with two groups resulting from scheduled mothers' club meetings and the other two from a gathering of street food sellers and their neighbours. Rowa-Dewar et al. (2008) used a similar approach by establishing 'open stalls', that is, stalls set at key locations around the community (i.e. library, church, etc.) where individuals could be asked about their views of cancer and cancer care.

The formation of groups can also be integrated into other methods of data collection. For instance, Ackerman et al. (2017) conducted informal focus groups in their study on the implementation of a new online patient portal in community health centres in California and they organised these groups while they carried out observations during staff tours of these medical facilities. The study was carried out over three months, but the researchers carried out intensive data collection for one day at each facility. The informal focus groups, instead of formal and previously scheduled focus groups, gave researchers the flexibility to incorporate these group discussions into other activities happening at the community health centres and other tasks performed by the research team (i.e. observations during staff tours).

Collecting Data in Focus Groups

We found that focus groups were particularly common in research carried out during complex health emergencies such as epidemics or natural disasters as this method allowed researchers to quickly capture the views of groups across multiple communities (Johnson and Vindrola-Padros et al., 2017). For instance, in a PRA that aimed to collect baseline information on community-based epidemic control priorities and identify strategies for containing Ebola in Liberia, Abramowitz et al. (2015) carried out 15 focus groups (n = 368) and observations (communities and emergency-response agencies) over a period of 20 days. The focus groups were facilitated by local field researchers in 15 communities and were made up of 15–20 participants of mixed gender (Abramowitz et al., 2015).

Another rapid study carried out during the 2014 Ebola outbreak also carried out focus groups, but included focus groups with healthcare workers' (HCWs) and pregnant and lactating women to explore their use of facilities during the epidemic (Dynes et al., 2015).

The focus group discussions were guided by a semi-structured topic guide that included questions on the use of health facilities for routine services, reasons for the decrease in use, perceptions of safety and recommendations to increase the use of facilities (Dynes et al., 2015). The focus group discussions were recorded in the form of notes and the research team analysed these by grouping them into common categories (Dynes et al., 2015).

I have used a similar technique when carrying out focus groups for rapid appraisals, where we have audio recorded the focus group discussions (in case we need additional information later in the in-depth analysis process) but have mainly taken detailed notes. We then transcribed the notes (normally taken by more than one researcher), compared the content across the researchers and identified the main findings. In some cases, each of the researchers has taken notes about all of the conversations. In other cases, where we have attempted to carry out the more targeted data collection, each researcher has focused on collecting data on a specific topic. Table 4.2 includes an example of a chart we have used to facilitate this process of dividing up topics for data collection. There was a natural overlap in some of the data collection, but this was addressed during the analysis as we carried out analysis as a team (see Chapter 5).

Table 4.2 Chart used for targeted data collection during focus groups

Topic	Main findings
Researcher 1	
Problems accessing facilities	
Problems within facilities	
Problems returning to facilities	
Problems accessing medication	
Researcher 2	
Strategies used to access facilities	
Strategies used to navigate care within facilities	
Strategies used to ensure continuity of care	
Strategies used to access medication	
Researcher 3	
Interventions/programmes delivered by the hospital to address problems accessing care	
Patient perceptions of these interventions/ programmes	

Another interesting approach for streamlining focus group discussions and analysis is the use of mind-maps proposed by Tattersall and Vernon (2007). Mind maps are developed as the focus group discussion is ongoing and are used to summarise the main topics discussed by the study participants. Participants are also asked to comment on the accuracy of the mind maps during the focus groups, adding a layer of 'member checking' to the process (Tattersall and Vernon, 2007).

Observations

In a review on the use of rapid ethnographies in healthcare, we found eight types of observations described by researchers (Vindrola-Padros and Vindrola-Padros, 2018). I outline each type and examples of studies that have used them in Table 4.3. These types of observations had different gradients of structure, ranging from completely unstructured to the use of structured observation guides. Unstructured observations normally rely on the collection of data in the form of fieldnotes in a field diary without maintaining any pre-established categories to organise these notes. The researcher freely records their observations and these are then transcribed and coded. Structured or semi-structured observations are based on the establishment of specific areas of observation before data collection begins. In the case of structured observations, these might even entail the filling out of a table or pro forma per observation episode to make sure all of the required data are collected.

Table 4.3 Types of observations described in a review on rapid ethnographies in healthcare (Vindrola-Padros and Vindrola-Padros, 2018)

Type of observation	Studies using this approach
Ethnographic observation	Chesluk et al. (2015); Mason et al. (2013); Saleem et al. (2015)
Video observations	Harte et al. (2016)
Participant observation	Choy et al. (2013); Coreil et al. (1989); Goepp et al. (2004); Hussain et al. (2015); Patmon et al. (2016)
Direct observation	Jayawardena et al. (2013); Murray et al. (2016); Needle et al. (2003)
Shadowing	Agyepong and Manderson (1994); Mullaney et al. (2012); Saleem et al. (2015)
Observations (type not specified)	Chesluk and Holmboe (2010); McElroy et al. (2007);
Tour observations	Ackerman et al. (2017)
Clinical observations	Wright et al. (2015)

When thinking about the suitability of observations for rapid qualitative research, I do not have any recommendations on which observation approach to use as both have proven valuable for rapid studies. Rapid ethnographies, for instance, have demonstrated that it is possible to carry out unstructured observations in a meaningful way during intensive and compressed periods of data collection. Armstrong and Armstrong (2018) combined different types of observations to collect data across multiple care homes over one-week fieldwork periods. They combined: (1) a general tour of the facilities, (2) observation shifts starting at 7:00 am and ending at midnight (to cover different times of the day), (3) observation shifts over weekdays and weekends (to cover different activities happening during the week), and (4) flash visit (one-day intensive field visit) at another care home in the locality to act as a comparator.

We have also integrated more 'dynamic' types of observation into our study as a way of gaining initial insight into an area or topic and then using this information to refine more in-depth forms of observation. These approaches have been labelled as 'touring', 'walk-along' or 'hanging out' methods. Ladner (2014) has argued that a tour of the area where the research will be carried out, whether this is a community, a hospital or an office, is a 'symbolic introduction' of the researcher to the location and those who will participate in the study. It might be the first exposure to the context and can act as an important data collection exercise. Notes from a tour would normally be taken in the form of unstructured observations and first impressions. In rapid qualitative studies, it can also function as a useful tool to organise subsequent, more in-depth observations, as the tour can be used to create an initial map of the areas, situations or events that need to be observed for the study.

Shadowing also entails some form of movement or tracking in the form of a tour, but is often used to understand the steps involved in a process or the stages of an individual's normal routine. Shadowing is used often in health services research to understand patient or staff experiences with a clinical pathway or their interactions with different areas of a hospital. Liberati (2017) has argued that shadowing in clinical settings can shed light on complex clinical activities such as information transfer and communication patterns that might have an impact on patient experience and care. In contrast to more static forms of observation, shadowing allows the researcher to capture and experience movement through areas and over time, thus presenting a more accurate representation of participants' experiences. It also allows the documentation of high volumes of data in short periods of time, which make it a method amenable to rapid qualitative research. We have normally limited shadowing sessions to two hours to prevent researcher and participant exhaustion (as having a 'shadow' can be intimidating) and a few of these sessions have normally been enough to get the required insight for a rapid study.

Hanging-out approaches are similar in the sense that they are loosely organised, but these might not entail movement in the form of a tour or shadowing. Hanging out involves being present in an area without a pre-established agenda and just letting yourself document what goes on around you (i.e. movements, informal conversations, body language, sounds and smells). Coffee break rooms, clinic waiting rooms, cafeterias and gardens are places where we have often used hanging-out approaches. These sessions can also be used to chat and build rapport with study participants. Rapid qualitative research often limits the amount of time we have available for the use of this observational method when compared to long-term ethnographic research. However, 'hanging-out' sessions can be purposively scheduled to document informal interactions in a given setting. In an interesting team-based rapid ethnography of a nursing care home, Armstrong and Lowndes (2018) combined different types of observations, including a tour of the care home as described earlier as well as observations in common areas, gardens and cafeterias where the researchers interacted with residents and staff. They have highlighted that these types of observations were important processes of data collection, but also made residents and staff more comfortable with their presence (Macdonald et al., 2018).

Some rapid qualitative research approaches such as RAPs have preferred more structured approaches to the collection of data through observations and have integrated structured observation guides into the field guides or manuals that I presented earlier in the chapter. The decision on which observation approach to use will depend on the research questions and the type of data required to answer these. I have found that structured observation guides have been particularly useful in studies where I am already familiar with the context (due to previous research) or in focused studies where I am seeking to collect detailed information. Examples of the latter include:

- Recording the information used to discuss patient cases in multidisciplinary team meetings
- Documenting how patients are referred to during hospital ward rounds
- Identifying instances when quality improvement is mentioned during hospital Board meetings
- Documenting the use of new medical technology (i.e. apps or other digital platforms) by healthcare workers

The structured guides I have used also vary in terms of their level of detail. Table 4.4 includes the categories used in the observation guides used for two studies. Both studies collected information in clinical settings, but the research questions guiding the studies required different types of information. Both studies also relied on the collection of data as a team, so the structured observation guides worked as a tool to ensure that all team members collected data in the same way.

Table 4.4 Comparison of structured observation guides used in two rapid qualitative studies

Example 1

	Pre-inspection brief	Inspection	Post-inspection debrief
Actors involved			

(Continued)

Table 4.4 (Continued)

Main activities	
Purpose of inspection	
Interaction of inspectors with ward nurses	
Interaction of inspectors with Multidisciplinary team	
Interaction of inspectors with patients	

Example 2	
Topic	*Notes*
General description of steps involved in patient journey	
Handovers between:	
- healthcare facilities	
- healthcare teams (same facility)	
along all sections of the pathway	
Factors acting as barriers to care or to good quality care	

Fieldnotes

Observations are documented in the form of fieldnotes. As mentioned earlier, note-taking can vary depending on how structured or unstructured these observations are. Fieldnotes can also vary in relation to the level of detail or completeness and type of data the researcher is documenting. The intensive data collection that is characteristic of most rapid qualitative studies means that researchers will probably not have enough time to collect detailed notes during an observation episode or while they are in the field. Researchers might then rely on the use of jottings or brief notes or a strategic selection of words that can act as a memory aide for the development of expanded notes that the researcher will then develop when they have left the field site or have some time to reflect and write (Vindrola-Padros, 2020).

In their iconic manual of RAP, Scrimshaw and Hurtado (1987) identify three types of information records that each researcher needs to maintain during the study: a brief diary (notes on what was done each day to act as a chronological record), brief fieldnotes (a few words on what was seen or heard), and expanded fieldnotes (on the same day, the researcher should expand on the brief fieldnotes and add comments and impressions in parentheses). The development of these expanded notes might also point to gaps in data collection that the researcher can document so this information can be collected the next day or at the next visit.

In addition to this process of fieldnote development, fieldnotes might also vary in relation to their purpose. Lowndes and Armstrong (2018) identified three types of field-notes developed by their team in a rapid ethnography:

- ***Substantive notes***: Describe situations and conversations with the aim of capturing as much detail as possible of what was observed.
- ***Reflective notes:*** Document the researcher's activities in the research setting, how they feel others see them and how their presence might change dynamics at their fieldsite.
- ***Analytic notes***: Begin the development of the interpretive work that will later be refined as all notes and other sources of data are analysed.

Mapping

Mapping has been used frequently in participatory research approaches such as participatory action research (PAR) and in rapid participatory approaches such as PRA. Mapping can be carried out by a researcher who is external to a community or area to obtain a sense of the spatial surroundings. Following more participatory approaches, it can also be used by community members to represent specific areas of their communities, identify problems and potential strategies to address these. In a previous book, we identified ways in which community-led mapping (referred to as perception mapping) was actively embraced by participants to identify areas in their communities where they thought cholera transmission would be more prevalent and the resources available to contain the spread of the epidemic (Whiteford and Vindrola-Padros, 2015). Hundt et al. (2004) used health walks with community members as one data collection method in their rapid ethnographic assessments (REA) on perceptions of stroke-like symptoms and health seeking behaviours in South Africa.

I have found mapping techniques useful when carrying out rapid qualitative research in organisations such as hospitals. In a recent study, we developed an approach for the rapid mapping of clinical pathways to identify barriers to care. The study lasted for three months, from set-up to the delivery of written findings. The mapping approach combined guided discussions with members of the clinical teams to develop an initial sketch of the pathway and data collection with patients and healthcare workers (HCWs) delivering care across the pathway to understand how these operated in practice. An observational 'shadowing technique' with HCWs and patients (as described earlier) was combined with semi-structured interviews. We used a structured observation guide to collect data during the shadowing. The initial sketch of the pathway was used as an elicitation device to generate discussion during the interviews. Table 4.5 includes a description of the different stages of the mapping process and the study timeline.

Table 4.5 Example of the use of rapid qualitative research to guide pathway process mapping

Stage	Timeline
Preparatory work	Week 1
• Process mapping outline	
• List of things to think about before meeting (types of pathways, general structure, things to consider in the study, potential barriers to data collection)	
Meeting 1: General mapping	Week 2
• Aims of the study	
• Outline of pathway mapping process	
• Impressions from research sites	
• Introduction to the rapid qualitative study design used for the mapping (work to be conducted in Months 2 and 3)	
Preparatory work/reading	
• Discuss and decide with teams what the pathways might look like	
• Decide who needs to attend Meetings 2 and 3 and invite them	
• Collect any information required for Meeting 2	
Meeting 2: First three pathways	Week 3
• Identification of pathway beginning and end for each procedure	
• Identification of 5–10 steps	
• Identification of knowledge gaps	
• General description of patient populations	
• Draft maps produced, to be refined through the next phase	

Stage	Timeline
Preparatory work/reading • Discuss with teams what the pathways might look like • Collect any information required for Meeting 3	
Meeting 3: Remaining two pathways • Identification of pathway beginning and end for each procedure • Identification of 5–10 steps • Identification of knowledge gaps • General description of patient populations • Draft maps produced, to be refined through the next phase	Week 4
Meeting 4 • Wrap up of pathway work not completed in Meetings 2 and 3 • Answer any questions/issues about the next stage – data collection and analysis (see below) • Agree plans for data collection	Week 5
Meeting 4b (if needed) Catch-up meeting with researchers • Answer any further questions/issues about the next stage – data collection and analysis	Week 6
Staff shadowing exercise for all pathways • Pathway in practice (how it is similar and differs from original map) • Potential problems, barriers, enablers • Relevant contextual factors • Analysis of data	Weeks 6–8
Patient shadowing exercise for all pathways • Pathway in practice (how it is similar and differs from original map) • Potential problems, barriers, enablers • Relevant contextual factors • Relevant patient characteristics shaping experiences with pathways	Weeks 8–10
Interviews with patients and staff (use of pathway maps as elicitation devices) • Confirm/expand the pathway maps • Identify additional barriers and enablers to access and deliver care • Document the local context	Weeks 6–10
Meeting 5 Analysis wrap-up meeting	Week 10
Final analysis and write-up	Weeks 11–12

The meetings set out for the development of the pathway sketch (Meetings 1–4) were facilitated by our research team through a series of pre-established questions, but the discussions were guided by the clinicians and managers who joined the meetings. The questions were organised across the different meetings and preparatory stages in the following ways.

Meeting 1: General Mapping

- When does the pathway start? When does it end?
- What story do we want our data to tell?
- What are the touchpoints during the patient's journey through the pathway?
- Who might be the key influencers, gatekeepers and decision-makers for each stage in the pathway (e.g. persons who may steer someone towards or away from health services)?
- What phases of the pathway create difficulties/encounter barriers?
- How can we improve these?

Preparatory Work/Reading before Meeting 2

Teams discuss the sketches for the pathways with relevant staff. They use these conversations to answer the following questions:

- Where does the pathway normally start and end?
- What are the different variations of the pathway?
- What are the handover points? (Points where patients or their information is handed over to another professional/organisation)
- Where are our knowledge gaps?
- Do we collect data on any stages of the pathway?
- Who is normally treated on the pathway? (Description of patient population)
- Who needs to be present during Meeting 2 to help map the pathway?

Prior to Meetings 2 and 3 the teams need to have sketched out a high level/outline map for each pathway, to be discussed and refined during the meeting.

Meeting 2: Three Pathways

The purpose of this meeting is to refine these four pathways. The main steps are:

1. Agree on pathway beginning and end.
2. Identify its main steps.
3. Indicate how much time each step takes.
4. Identify the main handover points.
5. Identify potential bottlenecks or other problems.
6. Identify the gaps in knowledge (These can be addressed during the data collection phase).

7 Describe the main patient populations.
8 Identify potential barriers in the delivery of care.

Preparatory Work/Reading before Meeting 3

The teams discuss the sketches for the pathways for two pathways with relevant staff. They use these conversations to answer the following questions:

- Where does the pathway normally start and end?
- What are the different variations of the pathway?
- What are the handover points? (Points where patients or their information is handed over to another professional/organisation)
- Where are our knowledge gaps?
- Do we collect data on any stages of the pathway?
- Who is normally treated on the pathway? (Description of patient population)
- Who needs to be present during Meeting 3 to help map the pathway?

Meeting 3: Two Pathways

The purpose of this meeting is to refine these two pathways. The steps are:

1. Agree on pathway beginning and end.
2. Identify its main steps.
3. Indicate how much time each step takes.
4. Identify the main handover points.
5. Identify potential bottlenecks or other problems.
6. Identify the gaps in knowledge (These can be addressed during the data collection phase).
7. Describe the main patient populations.
8. Identify potential barriers in the delivery of care.

Meeting 4

Wrap up pathway work not completed in Meetings 2 and 3.

As mentioned earlier, the outputs from Meetings 1–4 were sketches of pathways. These can then be developed into more 'user-friendly' representations of the pathway that can be used to elicit discussions during the interviews and guide the observations (see example in Figure 4.1). However, the conversations during these meetings were also useful for understanding the local context where care was delivered (including factors that could complicate delivery), variability in HCWs' views and potential barriers to care faced by patients.

C-SECTION PATHWAY

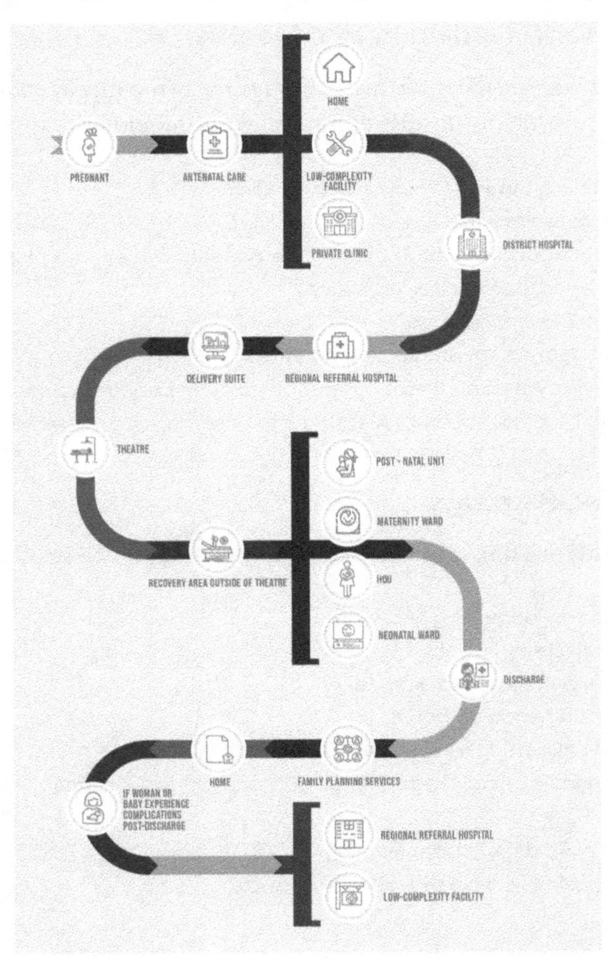

Visual abstract design: Franco Marquez

Figure 4.1 Example of user-friendly pathway diagram developed through collaborative meetings in a study aimed at the mapping of clinical pathways

Meeting 5

The teams bring the diagrams of the pathways sketched during Meetings 2–4 and the RAP sheets (or summaries) of data generated through the interviews and shadowing exercises. The discussions are guided by the following questions:

1. What are the stages of the pathway that the interviews and observations confirmed?
2. What are the stages of the pathway where there are discrepancies between the pathway maps and the collected data?
3. How can we use the interview and observation to enrich the pathway maps?
4. What are the different variations or types of patient journeys reflected in the interview and observation data? (We normally trace these variations on top of the pathway we sketched) Why are these variations produced?
5. What are the factors acting as barriers and enablers in patients' access to care?
6. What are the factors acting as barriers and enablers in the delivery of care?

Other researchers have combined similar techniques to the ones described earlier to map clinical pathways in rapid qualitative studies. Mullaney et al. (2012) carried out a quick ethnography to explore the experiences of patients undergoing radiotherapy treatment. The authors combined patient observations, informal interviews with staff, photographic documentation, and self-reported materials with patients to collect data on patient interactions and patients' emotional responses to these (Mullaney et al., 2012). The first phase of the study involved the main mapping activities. It lasted two weeks and relied on the use of observational methods to map the patient journeys across the hospital.

Visual Methods

Visual methods are now widely used in qualitative research as both alternative and complementary mechanisms to collect and generate data (Jones, 2004; Montgomery, 2009; Pfister et al., 2015; Roberts, 2000; Thomas and O'Kane, 1998). Some researchers have argued that visual methods in the form of photography, video, drawings, among others, have the capacity to maximise the involvement of a wider range of research participants, reduce power imbalances that are inherent to the research process and offer participants the opportunity to choose how they would like to express themselves (Barker and Weller, 2003; Crivello et al., 2009; Johnson, 2011; Luttrell, 2010; Mitchell, 2006; Thomas and O'Kane, 2000; Vindrola-Padros, 2012; Young and Barret, 2001).

Visual methods have also played an important role in rapid qualitative research as some authors have argued that intensive periods of data collection can be facilitated through the use of video or photography. For instance, Pink and Morgan (2013) included video as one way to ensure that researchers are able to capture in-depth data over short periods of fieldwork when carrying out short-term ethnographies. According to them, videos facilitate the rapid capturing of large volumes of data (i.e. conversations, interactions, body language, etc.) for in-depth analysis that can take place after the fieldwork is over (Pink and Morgan, 2013).

In an application of this approach, Harte et al. (2016) combined video footage, observational fieldnotes, and post-natal video-cued interviews to guide in-depth analysis focused on exploring the hospital design factors influencing childbirth supporters' experiences. The video footage facilitated the in-depth analysis of one family's experience of childbirth and was used to guide discussions during interviews, while acting as a 'member checking' process. The use of video in this study allowed researchers to capture the complexity of the experiences of birth supporters and how these were shaped by the built environment within a short timeframe.

Other visual methods such as photography have been extensively discussed in the literature and could also be adapted for rapid studies (Ewald, 2000; Hubbard, 1994; Wang, 1999). My primary experience with the use of visual methods in rapid qualitative research is based on the use of different types of drawing and 'draw and write' techniques with adult and child research participants. These techniques can include processes where research participants are shown images to prompt discussion on topics, or are asked to create original drawings and, in some cases, also provide an explanation of the image (e.g. see; Backett-Milburn et al., 2003; Curtis et al., 2004; Johnson et al., 2012; Mitchell, 2006: 61–62; Pelander et al., 2007; Vindrola-Padros, 2012).

Drawings with Staff

I have found drawings helpful for quickly documenting the role people play within teams, departments or organisations. In a rapid ethnography documenting the role of a non-governmental organisation (NGO) in the delivery of support to families whose children were receiving cancer treatment in Argentina, I used a drawing technique to understand how individuals viewed the organisation where they worked and their working relationships with other NGO staff. The session with each study participant included the following steps:

1. I explained the structure of the session and the reason why I had decided to use drawings.
2. I gave the participant a few blank pages and coloured pencils to make the drawing. I instructed them to draw themselves and then draw the members of staff they worked with more frequently, closer to them and those they rarely worked with, farther away. Participants were not asked to discuss the drawing as they were making it, but many chose to do so.
3. After the participant finished the drawing, I asked them to explain it to me and started a formal interview about their history within the NGO, the NGO's strategy and the support they offered to families. We often went back to the drawings in many of the interviews, using these as an elicitation device to facilitate the conversation.

I implemented this drawing technique, interviews with staff and structured observations during team meetings and routine delivery of services to families over a three-month period. The drawings were an easy and quick way to elicit in-depth data on complex and multi-factorial working relationships. For most of the participants, the drawings were an enjoyable experience; they functioned as an icebreaker and eliminated the formality of the session.

Drawings with Patients and Family Members

I have also found drawings helpful as a mechanism for documenting patients' journeys and their experiences of diagnosis and treatment. In a rapid qualitative study with children receiving cancer treatment in Argentina, I used the 'draw and write technique' to capture their experiences of leaving their home to obtain cancer treatment in a distant city (for a detailed description of the study and drawing process see Johnson et al., 2012). The session with the children involved the creation of three different types of drawings and I used the drawings to guide the discussion through an interview. The children were asked to complete:

- A freestyle drawing where they were asked to draw anything they liked. This drawing allowed them to feel comfortable with the method and it gave them the opportunity to identify and discuss new issues that I had not previously considered.
- Diagnosis and treatment scenes. The instructions were left vague on purpose to see what events, people, and objects children associated with these stages (see examples of these drawings in Figure 4.2).
- A third drawing of their most difficult and happy moments. Here, the idea was to see if these drawings were associated with any particular part of the medical treatment.

In the same study, I also used the drawing technique during the interviews I conducted with the children's parents. The drawing session with the parents was organised around the creation of a visual life course timeline where they were instructed to draw the different stages of their life. They were free to choose the format of their timeline and were allowed to include writing. All of the parents included the child's cancer diagnosis and treatment in their timelines. I used the drawing of the timeline to construct parents' journeys and narratives of diagnosis and treatment.

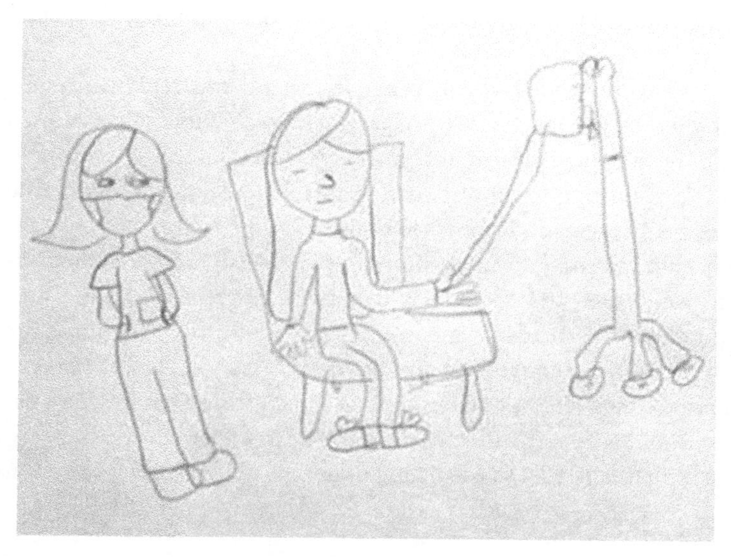

Figure 4.2 Examples of children's drawings of cancer treatment

Listing, Sorting and Rating

Some rapid qualitative studies have used techniques that rely on participants making lists, or grouping and ranking items. Techniques such as pile sorting and free listing are not new and have often been used in quantitative research. Certain adaptations of these approaches have been made by qualitative researchers seeking to obtain data from study participants in a timely way. These types of approaches have also been identified as participatory methods in the sense that they allow the participant to lead data generation sessions and can also be used by field researchers without previous research experience (useful for studies where community members are empowered to become researchers themselves) (Trotter et al., 2001).

Free listing includes asking participants to make a list based on instructions or prompts made by the researcher. Trotter et al. (2001) have argued that free listing has three main uses:

1. Create a list of salient topics that can then be used to develop questions in an interview.
2. Combine lists to explore variation in a particular domain.
3. Determine individual and group limits of knowledge about a particular domain.

When using rapid assessment, response and evaluation model (RARE), for instance, researchers have used free listing as an initial component of focus groups. Trotter et al. (2001) asked study participants to list all of the different people they felt would be most vulnerable to human immunodeficiency virus (HIV) infection in their community. They then asked them to organise the people in four groups and order them by degree of vulnerability (1 most vulnerable to 4 as the least vulnerable). They proceeded with the focus group questions and asked participants to identify the conditions in their communities that made people vulnerable to Acquired Immune Deficiency Syndrome (AIDS), organisations in the community that provided support, and existing and new interventions.

Free lists can be used as a way to generate insight into a particular topic that can then be explored in greater depth through interviews or focus group discussions, but the process of developing lists can also be analysed as a source of information. Daley et al. (2012) used free listing to capture participants' perceptions of local barriers to colon cancer screening. Participants were asked to list all of the factors that they thought operated as barriers to screening in their community. The lists were then analysed based on which items were listed first (assuming that those of greatest salience are mentioned first), the number of participants mentioning the item, the total number of items on individual lists and the common order of the items (Daley et al., 2012).

Weller and Romney (1988) have argued that free listing exercises vary depending on the types of questions asked by the interviewer. The interviewer can ask a very open question that can potentially lead to the listing of dozens of items, they can ask for a limited list (name the top five items), or can ask the participant to reflect on multiple lists at the same time (i.e. disease terms and symptoms and causes of each disease).

Pile sorting can involve asking participants to group items developed through free listing as in the example mentioned earlier or researchers can use previously developed cards that participants will need to group based on their instructions. In this type of task, the aim is for participants to sort the cards into piles that are more similar to each other than they are to cards in separate piles (Weller and Romney, 1988). This task can be constrained (participants are told the number of piles they can create) or unconstrained (they can create as many piles as they wish). The sorting process can be divided into different types:

- ***Single sorting***: Participants are provided with the cards and given instructions on how to sort them into piles.
- ***Successive sorting***: Sorting can also entail a series of sorting instructions to allow participants to create classification trees or taxonomies (sorting items into piles and then asking how they would subdivide those piles into smaller groups).
- ***Triadic comparisons***: Participants are asked to compare items in groups of three.
- ***Rating scales***: Participants are asked to order items in one or multiple scales based on pre-established criteria.
- ***Matching***: Participants are provided with two lists or two piles of items and are asked to match the items based on specific instructions (Weller and Romney, 1988).

In previous research, we have used these approaches as tools to generate data for a study, but have also used them during the early stages of study design to elicit the views of the study stakeholders. As mentioned in Chapter 3, when co-designing a rapid qualitative study, we would normally have one or more meetings or workshops with stakeholders. These would normally be used to identify the reasons why a study is required, the areas that need to be covered and the time points when study findings need to be shared. In a recent study, we worked with stakeholders to design a rapid evaluation of a programme aimed at delivering support to parents whose children had learning disabilities. The budget and time for the evaluation were limited and we needed to make sure the evaluation was focused enough to provide robust findings. We met with the stakeholder group on two occasions. The first meeting was guided by a free listing exercise where the attendees listed the core elements of the programme and were asked to group them in three different ways: (1) in order of importance to the organisation delivering the programme, (2) in order of importance to those receiving the support, (3) considering how urgent evaluation findings would be in relation to their effectiveness. We then collected all of the information and analysed it to generate average rankings for the whole group of attendees. The second meeting was used to discuss these results and use them to design the scope and research questions guiding the rapid evaluation.

Documentary Analysis

Most of the rapid qualitative studies we have carried out to date have involved at least one aspect of documentary analysis. By documents we are referring to reports, meeting agendas and minutes, leaflets, educational posters or other materials for users and text-based content on websites that are relevant to the study. We have reviewed documents with the following aims:

- ***Familiarisation with the topic and/or context under study before the study begins:*** In rapid qualitative research, preparation is everything as the time for data collection in the field is limited. Documents developed on the topic, intervention, community or service we will be studying will be useful to contextualise researchers before beginning with the fieldwork.
- ***Capture changes over time:*** Rapid qualitative research can only capture a snapshot of a process or situation. Documents are useful in helping to create a retrospective picture that can then be used to inform data collection in real-time.
- ***Include discussions or situations in a study that we cannot observe first-hand:*** Here I am referring particularly to the analysis of documents such as meeting minutes or notes. If researchers are not able or allowed to carry out observations during these meetings, meeting notes or minutes (although not the same as being there) can act as a proxy and give the team insight into the nature of the discussions during these meetings. These can then be triangulated with the data we can collect at these sites, such as data generated through interviews.
- ***Analyse the 'official' story versus what happens in practice:*** The description of programmes, services or interventions in official documents can be used to identify assumptions behind how these were designed or their intended outcomes. These 'official versions' can then be compared with data we might have collected on how their implementation played out in practice.
- ***Compare with other sites, individuals, programmes where we cannot collect primary data:*** As mentioned earlier, rapid qualitative research needs to pay close attention to sampling as data collection needs to be targeted to be completed in a short amount of time. In previous studies, we have used documents developed by other sites or services to compare these data with the data we generated in our research sites. In this way, these documents helped us develop some 'loose comparators' where we might not have the same depth of data as in the case of our research sites, but can at least have an idea of situations or issues in other locations.

Rapid documentary analysis includes the steps outlined in Table 4.6. It is presented as a linear process in this table for the sake of simplicity, but, in practice, this is an iterative process that involves extracting data from documents and then going back to look for missing documents or information and beginning the process all over again. We normally carry out documentary analysis in parallel to other forms of data collection and analysis with interview data and observation data. The documentary analysis might also be used to address gaps in knowledge identified through the other research methods.

Table 4.6 Steps involved in documentary analysis

Step	Description
1. Design	Define the aims, topics/areas to be covered, dates of the documents and develop a sampling framework to guide the collection of documents
2. Document selection	Select the documents that match the inclusion/exclusion criteria and create a document inventory (we normally do this on a spreadsheet and maintain a shared digital file of all documents)
3. Data extraction	We use a pro forma or data extraction form to obtain the necessary information from the documents. This can also be done through the use of a spreadsheet, but we have also used, shared electronic forms and online questionnaires such as those created on Research Electronic Data Capture (REDCap)
4. Data synthesis	We analyse all extracted data and synthesise it based on the aims of the documentary analysis and our research questions
5. Triangulation	We integrate the findings of the documentary analysis with the data generated through other methods of data collection

Structured Approaches: Field Manual and Field Guides

In order to speed up the process of data collection and to ensure consistency in data collection across multiple field researchers, several rapid qualitative approaches use field manuals or field guides. RAPs and REAs were the first to experiment with these approaches and relied on the use of tables or forms that could be used to collect data from interviews, observations or focus groups. In some cases, research teams have developed full manuals for researchers composed of study background information, tables or forms for data collection, topics to discuss during team debriefings and a field site itinerary. Table 4.7 has an example of the contents included in a field guide used by McMullen et al. (2011) to explore the implementation of clinical decision support in community hospital settings.

The process for developing field guides or manuals varies and these are normally informed by some of the work carried out during the preparatory and scoping phases described in Chapter 3. Hurtado (1990) has also developed a process for piloting field guides where a focus group is organised with field researchers and, after they have gone through the content in the field guide, they are asked questions such as those following Table 4.7.

Table 4.7 Information and forms included in a field guide used for a RAP (McMullen et al., 2011)

Site visit preparation schedule
Site profile instrument
Sample site visit schedule
Sample fact sheet
Sample interview guide
Sample fieldnotes form
Sample field survey instrument
Agenda for team debriefings

- Can you understand each page of the field guide easily?
- Can you readily identify what you are being asked to do?
- Do you think you can perform what you are being asked to do?
- Do you think the field guide is for someone like you or for someone else?
- Would you make any changes to the guide?

The field guide is revised based on the answers to these questions and focus group participants can also be asked to draw pictures in relation to the content in the field guide, so these can be integrated as an additional explanatory tool (Hurtado, 1990). In our experience, balance needs to be reached between maintaining the flexibility of the guides (to make changes as data collection is ongoing) and making sure all researchers adhere to the norms and structure set-out in the guide (and rapidly inform the team if changes are required). Frequent team meetings are helpful for discussing and agreeing potential changes that might need to be made to the guide.

Chapter Summary

- Data collection methods used frequently in qualitative research such as interviews, focus groups, observations and documentary analysis can be adapted to rapid study designs.
- Most of these adaptations rely on focusing the scope of data collection to cover more ground, carrying out data collection and analysis in parallel, intensifying data collection to capture greater volumes of data, and using structured tools to maintain the focus of the research and ensure consistency in data collection across researchers.
- A rapid interviewing technique developed by my team includes the taking of notes during interviews, the synthesis of these notes in a table (called a RAP sheet) and the use of this table to share emerging findings with other members of the team and relevant stakeholders.
- Researchers have reduced the amount of time required for focus groups by recruiting participants in natural or existing groups, using structured tools to collect data and carrying out mapping exercises or other forms of data analysis and interpretation as the groups are ongoing.
- Researchers using observations as a data collection method can develop different types of notes (jottings, longer notes, interpretive notes) depending on the aims of the study and can use structured observation guides to facilitate the targeted focus of observations and consistency across researchers.
- Some authors have argued that visual methods facilitate the intensive collection of data over short amounts of time.
- Rapid review techniques (for searching, extracting and synthesis) are helpful when carrying out documentary analysis in the context of rapid research.

Discussion Questions

1. Select one of the data collection methods discussed in the chapter and identify the ways in which it can be adapted for rapid qualitative research designs.
2. What are some of the problems researchers might encounter while making these adaptations?
3. Are there other data collection methods that could be used in rapid studies that are not included in the chapter? How could these be adapted to short study timeframes?

Exercise 4

What is the Best Data Collection Method for this Research Question?

Option A

Think about your own study. Considering the research questions and rapid qualitative research approach you developed for Exercise 3, identify the best data collection methods for your study. Use the following table to help you map the methods, the data you aim to collect and how the data will help you answer your research question.

Research questions (RQs)	Data collection methods	Type of data you think you will obtain using this method	How will you use these data to answer the research question?
RQ 1			
RQ 2			
...			

Option B

Using the research questions you developed for the case study in Exercise 3, identify the best data collection methods for your study. Use the following table to help you map the methods, the data you aim to collect and how the data will help you answer your research question.

Research questions (RQs)	Data collection methods	Type of data you think you will obtain using this method	How will you use these data to answer the research question?
RQ 1			
RQ 2			
...			

Case study: Programme to support parents of children with learning disabilities

A new programme aimed at supporting parents of children with learning disabilities is being rolled out across three neighbourhoods through their local community centres. Your team has been asked to develop a rapid qualitative study with the aim of documenting the process of implementation and capture lessons learnt that could be used to inform the rollout of the programme in other neighbourhoods.

Your team is composed of three full-time researchers. The study should not last more than six months and emerging findings need to be shared two months after the study start date to inform decisions that need to be made during the early implementation phase.

5

DATA ANALYSIS AND INTERPRETATION

Rapid qualitative research creates interesting challenges to traditional ways of doing qualitative research. Most rapid qualitative research approaches tend to view data collection and analysis as processes that need to take place in parallel, continuously informing each other. In this book, I chose to describe data collection and analysis in separate chapters for simplicity, but both chapters make reference to how these processes intertwine. This chapter places an emphasis on the approaches commonly used in rapid qualitative research to analyse data, identifying ways in which researchers have modified these for short study timeframes.

Analysis Begins in the Field

Rapid qualitative research tends to use an approach for data analysis composed of the following stages: (1) debriefing and synthesis of emerging findings while still in the field, (2) data reduction (can also start in the field), (3) data interpretation, and (4) data visualisation or representation (Beebe 2014; Sangaramoorthy and Kroeger, 2020; Scrimshaw and Hurtado, 1987). When carrying out data collection, rapid qualitative researchers tend to develop brief summaries of data, sometimes as frequently as on a daily basis. Rapid research teams will also meet frequently to discuss emerging findings, so data analysis begins almost at the same time as data are collected. Data are also organised while in the field, with different aspects of translation and perhaps even some selected transcription of audio recordings happening during data collection to begin sorting data into manageable formats. In the case of researchers using visual data, photographs or drawings might also be selected or at least categorised during fieldwork (Halme et al., 2016; Ladner, 2014). After this initial sorting and summarising, rapid qualitative researchers will often use some of the techniques for data reduction, interpretation and representation outlined in the following sections.

Table-Based Methods

Tables and matrices are my favourite way of reducing data. These are frequently used in rapid qualitative research to provide a brief overview of the data (data display technique) as well as to compare findings across sites, cases or researchers (see Table 5.1). Some authors have argued that rapid assessment procedures (RAPs) are adequate for the rapid collection of data but demand more time during the analysis (Holdsworth et al., 2020). This overlooks the main characteristics of RAPs in relation to their iterative design (data collection and analysis are carried out in parallel) and the use of tables or templates to aid the rapid cataloguing and synthesis of data.

As indicated in Chapter 4, I have used RAP sheets as a way of summarising findings while carrying out data collection, but have also used RAP sheets during the early stages of data analysis after data collection is complete. RAP sheets bring together the main findings collected through interviews, observations, documents and other methods.

RAP sheets can be as simple and short or as long as research teams need them to be. If using them to share emerging findings while carrying out data collection, I would recommend that RAP sheets be kept short and findings summarised as much as possible (especially if data are collected by a large group of field researchers). In a more in-depth data analysis phase at the end of the study, however, researchers can go back to the original RAP sheets and start adding more detail to the findings and even illustrative quotes if the voice recordings have been analysed and/or transcribed. The tabular format is still used to organise the findings, but it will contain more detail.

The RADaR technique has been proposed as a different way of transforming textual data into more user-friendly formats (Watkins, 2017). The RADaR technique requires that all data are transcribed and that these transcripts use the same format. The data are then copied and pasted onto a master table capturing some basic information of the interviewee, but mainly including the interview questions and the interviewee responses (Watkins 2017). The table can also include an additional column, so the researcher can make some notes reflecting on the data. If the analysis is carried out by an individual researcher, they will then reflect on the main findings from this table they would like to focus on in the next stage. If doing the analysis as part of a team, the team would then meet to discuss the first table to discuss what would be included in the second stage, which involves a more specific table. This process of moving to a second table involves a process of focusing and elimination of data and this selection process is based on the data the researchers feel will help them answer the research questions guiding the study. The reviewing and discussion (in the case of team-based analysis) will be repeated to make decisions in relation to what to include in a third table. This process of reduction can continue until the researcher/s have decided that the information included in the table is enough to help them answer the research question/s and the extent to which they have identified the data they need to explain the main findings of the study (normally in the form of quotes from interview transcripts or snippets from observation notes) (Watkins, 2017).

Table 5.1 Table-based methods for data analysis in rapid qualitative research

Method	Description	Process of reduction	Examples of studies
Rapid assessment procedure (RAP) sheets	Use of tables to summarise findings as data collection is ongoing and to guide initial stages of analysis after data collection is complete.	Reduce data being generated through multiple methods to a bullet point list of the most important findings. This list can then be expanded through a second round of analysis.	Beebe (2001) first proposed the use of RAP sheets to summarise study findings, but we have adapted their use to include the steps described in this chapter (Vindrola-Padros et al. 2020).
RADaR technique	Reduction of text-based data through multiple processes of data reduction cycles where data are organised from general to specific tables.	Reduce all text-based data to a selection of data that can be used to answer the research questions.	Watkins (2017)
Paraphrasing table	Use of tables or 'data cards' to move from direct quotes of the data to summaries based on paraphrasing what participants said.	Organisation of raw data into categories. Summarise the main points expressed in the raw data. Develop participant data cards and establish a coherent metaphor.	Ladner (2014)
Framework analysis	Raw data are organised in a table where the cases (participants, observation episodes, etc.) are organised according to rows and the main topics or categories are organised in the columns.	Raw data are organised according to pre-established categories as well as new ones emerging from the data. Categories are grouped in larger themes.	Keith et al. (2017) Gale et al. (2013)
Template-based method	A pre-established template (informed by the research questions and the literature) is used to synthesise the data.	Transcripts or other forms of text are summarised using a pre-established template. A matrix is then created with the data from the template.	Taylor et al. (2018) Gale et al. (2019)

Framework analysis has been used frequently in team-based health services research. One of the approaches that I have found helpful to adapt for rapid qualitative research is the one developed by Gale et al. (2013). This approach involves the following steps:

Step 1: Transcription.
Step 2: Familiarisation with the interview by reading through the transcripts and recording any thoughts or impressions in the form of notes.
Step 3: Coding the interview transcript by applying a label or code that can be used to describe the interpretation of the raw data.

Step 4: After initial coding, members of the team get together to discuss the codes they have used so far and agree on a codebook or analytical framework.
Step 5: The analytical framework is then applied consistently across all transcripts.
Step 6: A spreadsheet is then used to chart the coded data, where the cases (or interview transcripts) are organised in the rows and the codes are situated in the columns. These codes can be grouped in larger categories, if appropriate.
Step 7: Characteristics and differences across the data are identified, creating connections, looking at the data through lenses created by different theoretical frameworks, and developing typologies (Gale et al., 2013).

At the end of this chapter, I describe how I have combined the use of RAP sheets with framework analysis to facilitate rapid qualitative data analysis.

Thematic Analysis

A recent review on the use of rapid ethnographies in healthcare highlighted that the most common data analysis method was thematic analysis (Vindrola-Padros and Vindrola-Padros, 2018). In some cases, the use of thematic analysis in these studies followed the same steps as in long-term research, which include: familiarisation with the data, assigning preliminary codes to the data, searching for patterns between codes and revising initial codes, grouping codes into wider themes, defining and naming themes and describing themes in the text with the use of examples from the data (Braun and Clarke, 2006; Nowell et al., 2017).

Some rapid studies, however, have made minor modifications or adaptations to increase the speed of analysis. As mentioned earlier, Keith et al. (2017) used the period of data collection to familiarise themselves with the data and map out their approach for analysis. This allowed them to reduce the amount of time they needed to develop the initial codes. Ash et al. (2010) divided the interview transcripts and fieldnotes between different members of the team, not carrying out full double coding of the data, but implementing a limited degree of cross-checking between researchers. Taylor et al. (2018) followed a similar approach when adapting thematic analysis to a rapid design, carrying out full double coding for some transcripts but not for the entire dataset.

The Codebook

Many rapid qualitative studies have relied on the use of a codebook or code manual to guide the coding process (particularly those coding as a team). According to Crabtree and Miller, 'the code manual is a data management tool; it is used to organise segments of similar or related text for ease in interpretation and to search for confirming/disconfirming evidence of these interpretations' (1999: 167). Codebooks normally have the following sections: the code, a brief definition, a full definition, guidelines for when to use the code, guidelines for when not to use the code and examples (MacQueen et al., 1998).

The codebook is iterative and can be modified throughout the data analysis and writing processes (Crabtree and Miller, 1999). Table 5.2 includes an example of a codebook we developed for a rapid qualitative study.

Table 5.2 Example of a codebook used in a rapid qualitative study (Chisnall et al., under review)

Code	Description	Example of its application
General data-use	General comments/ opinions regarding qualitative data-use	'I'm very aware that we tend to look at data and focus very much on, on numbers and quantitative data, and yet a massive amount of data comes through narrative and stories and that can be really, really influential and informative, um even in what you might think of as more sort of black and white quantitative times. So I think we neglect to use that sort of data, um enough and that we don't sort of maybe use it to create patterns of, of ways of thinking about a problem, and to really listen to those that are being affected by the problem'. – PAR 14
Unrealised communication potential	Where individuals express the opinion that communication needs to be increased	'I do think that is definitely something we as social scientists need to be a bit more strategic about' – PAR 01
Realised communication potential	Where individuals express the opinion that information communication has been achieved with positive outcome	'Yes it's working, because I feel like a lot of us actually look forward to that email every single night, because we might not know anything about what is going on in the hospital, because we don't actually go, so we're not physically present there, but just by receiving those emails, it just kind of tells us that we are an important person, to the hospital in general. That's why they're sending out these emails, so that we are on the same page as they are. So, it's kind of something that gives us a lot of positivity at the end of the day, prompts us to go back to work, because a lot of us are like, we're like we are so done with working from home, that we just want to go back, so yes'. – PAR 11
Information hierarchy	A system in which members of an organisation or society are ranked according to relative status or authority	'Yeah, I mean there are these trees, these sort of like, you know, um, what you, you know, sort of that tree of hierarchy of who's in what role and like how they sort of tend to disseminate information' – PAR 08

The development of a codebook is an iterative process, but the following steps have been identified:

1. Develop initial code list (before or after data collection).
2. Circulate the proposed list for review.
3. Develop detailed code definitions.
4. Coders independently code the same text.
5. Assess the consistency of code application.

6 In the case of codes that are acceptable and consistent, continue coding.
7 In the case of codes that are unacceptable and inconsistent, revise the codebook.
8 Recode all previously coded text with the unacceptable codes using the new guidelines (MacQueen et al., 1998).

Codebooks have benefits and limitations. Codebooks have been used frequently in studies where research teams have to share emerging findings on a regular basis and are pressured to deliver these early on in the study. Ash et al. (2012) developed 'rough themes' during data collection using a type of codebook. This approach allowed them to share emerging findings at each of the sites where they collected data. It was also helpful in establishing a member-checking process, where participants were asked to comment on the research team's interpretation and presentation of the data (Ash et al., 2012; see also Patmon et al., 2016).

Codebooks can be used to code data generated from interviews or focus groups, but can also be developed to incorporate data generated from observations and content from documentary analysis. Saleem et al. (2015) for instance, used the same codebook to code fieldnotes from observations and data from the interviews and argued that this approach facilitated triangulation and the generation of a thick description of the barriers and facilitators to the use of clinical information systems in intensive care units.

Codebooks that are developed in advance or during early stages of data collection allow researchers to start with data analysis while data collection is ongoing. The codebooks can be changed throughout the study as new findings emerge. Despite these benefits, studies that establish codes before data collection or before data collection is complete, run the risk of setting pre-established categories to look at the data that might blind the researcher from findings they had not anticipated. Shaw et al. (2016) propose an in-between approach, deciding on some codes a priori, but adding codes during and after data collection. Teams also have to make decisions in relation to the level of detail that will be included in the codebook, running the risk of having a codebook where codes are so broad that they could be used to code significant amounts of text or so specific that they miss out relevant information (Crabtree and Miller, 1999).

Other Forms of Visualisation

RAPs and rapid appraisals are known for their reliance on data visualisation as a way of generating early interpretations as well as tools for the cross-checking of these interpretations with study participants (Beebe, 2001; Scrimshaw and Hurtado, 1987). Data visualisation entails the translation of recorded or text-based data into graphical form. Qualitative data can also be quantified, but I have focused only on graphical representations of qualitative data that maintain its qualitative aspect. Some of the commonly used graphic representations include:

- ***Organisational charts:*** To show the relationships between people or areas of an organisation (Scrimshaw and Hurtado, 1987)
- ***Flow charts or process maps:*** To illustrate the series of steps involved in a process or contrast the flow of events
- ***Causal networks or social maps:*** To show the relationships between people, events or locations (Sangaramoorthy and Kroeger, 2020)
- ***Taxonomies:*** Grouping data according to pre-established categories or families
- ***Cognitive or mind maps:*** Synthesise perceptions or ways of thinking about a particular topic and the interrelationship between its different components (Tattersall and Vernon, 2007)

When carrying out rapid evaluations, one of the first things we do is develop a programme theory, a description of the aims, main activities and expected outcomes of the intervention as well as the mechanisms the intervention designers and implementers thought the intervention would need to achieve these outcomes (see Davidoff et al., 2015 for examples of programme theories). We have found that diagrams such as the one included in Figure 5.1 are one of the most effective ways of visualising this information and using it to make interpretations in relation to the assumptions made when developing the intervention.

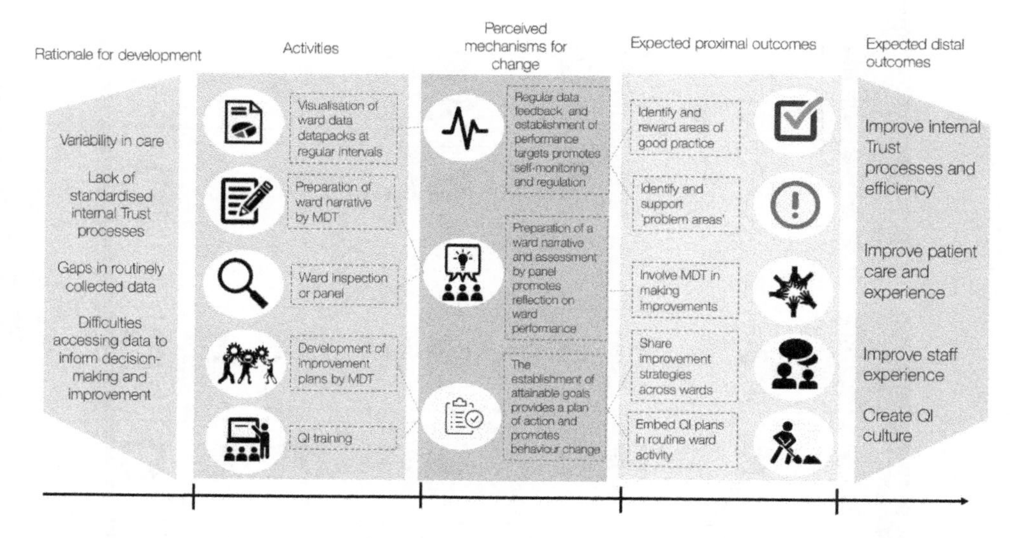

Figure 5.1 Programme theory developed for a programme process evaluation

We have also used diagrams in rapid evaluations to identify the degree to which an intervention has been rolled out in the same way across multiple sites. Figure 5.2, for instance, shows the number of activities that formed part of the intervention and the extent to which these were carried out across ten hospital wards. The data were collected in the form of interview transcripts with hospital staff and observations during team meetings

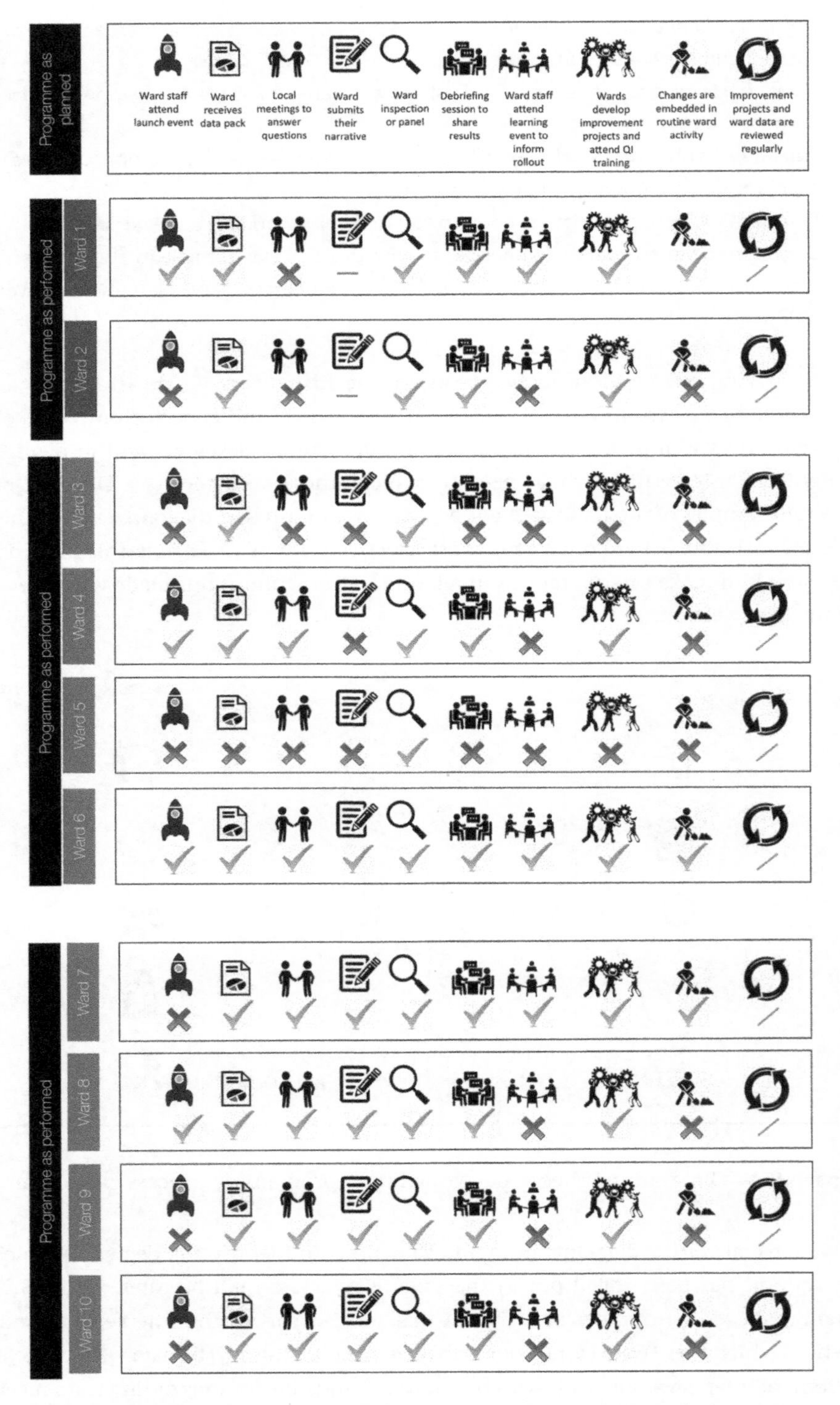

Figure 5.2 Implementation of the programme across wards

and other meetings related to the implementation of the programme. We asked staff about the involvement of the ward in the activities and searched for evidence of these in our observation notes. It wasn't until we mapped these data in the diagram in Figure 5.2 that we were able to see that not all wards had access to the same types of activities that formed part of the intervention. As the intervention was rolled out in a staggered way, we were also able to see that implementation improved as the rollout progressed in the sense that the wards that received the intervention towards the end of the rollout period had access to more of the activities than the wards that received it during early stages.

Member Checking

Several rapid qualitative studies have incorporated member checking (where participants are sent the findings of a study and can provide feedback on the researchers' interpretations) as a form of validation of the interpretations made by the researchers. In some cases, this was carried out when the final analysis was complete, but before the submission of a final report (Patmon et al., 2016). In these cases, study participants were sent a draft of the final analysis or given a presentation of the main findings and were asked to provide feedback (Patmon et al., 2016). In other cases, the member checking process was incorporated into the data collection methods as in the case of the use of mind maps during focus groups mentioned earlier (Tattersall and Vernon, 2007), where study participants could see the researcher's interpretation and main synthesis of the findings and provide feedback in real time.

The level of formality of member checking processes varies and some consider these interactions with participants as an active stage in the research process. In their focused ethnography on perceptions of falls in the elderly, Kilian et al. (2008) presented the member checking process as a form of data elaboration, instead of only verification. This was done with a sub-sample of the study participants who took part in an interview that was carried out after preliminary analyses were completed. These interviews were used to explore topics in greater depth (Kilian et al., 2008).

Rapid Data Analysis Process Combining the RAP Sheet and Framework Analysis

As mentioned at the beginning of the chapter, the process of data analysis begins as data are being collected. RAP sheets are one way to begin the process of synthesising study findings and identifying the key topics or areas of focus for the team. Figure 5.3 includes a description of a process of data analysis that can be carried out after at least some data have been added to the RAP sheet. This process includes the following steps:

1. Review the RAP sheet to identify emerging topics that need to be explored in further detail.
2. Arrange the research team in sub-groups (if possible) with a lead to manage this additional analytical work.
3. Develop an outline of the analysis informed by a review of relevant literature, theoretical frameworks that might be useful and key issues emerging from the data.
4. Organise the team to go back to the raw data and carry out full or selective transcription of interview recordings or fieldnotes.
5. Develop a coding framework and discuss it within the wider team.
6. Code the data and chart it using the framework analysis method (see earlier in the chapter).
7. Explore relationships and patterns in the charted data.

These more in-depth analyses can then be described in short reports, presentation slides or visual materials such as infographics. They can also be developed into individual manuscripts for publication. I discuss different avenues for dissemination in Chapter 7.

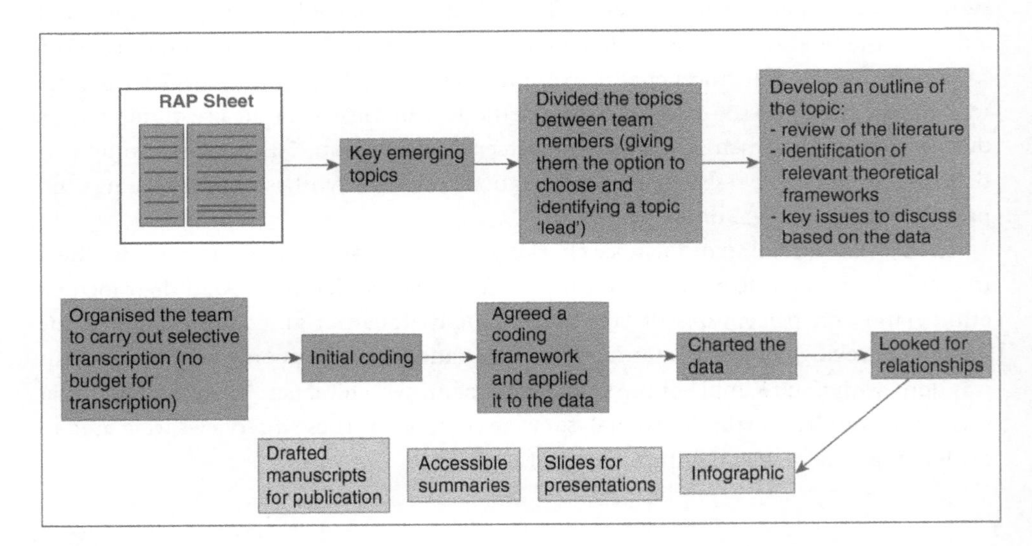

Figure 5.3 Rapid qualitative analysis process combining the RAP sheet and framework analysis

Chapter Summary

- Analysis begins in the field as teams might synthesise findings and have debriefing meetings during data collection.
- Rapid qualitative studies have relied on table or template-based methods as a way of categorising data quickly, facilitating team-based analysis, triangulating data from multiple sources and enabling cross-case comparisons.

- Researchers need to be careful with the use of pre-established templates for data analysis as these might not allow the identification of new topics emerging from the data (not originally considered by the researcher).
- Team-based data analysis can be facilitated by the use of a codebook to ensure all researchers are coding data in the same way.
- Several authors have described the use of different types of data visualisation techniques (charts, process maps, trees or taxonomies) as a way of generating early interpretations of the data.
- Member checking, where research participants are able to review emerging findings and provide feedback, can help the research team to cross-check their interpretations of the data.

Discussion Questions

1 What are the main table-based data analysis methods for rapid qualitative research described in the chapter?
2 What are the strengths and limitations of table-based methods?
3 What are some of the approaches for rapid data analysis that are not mentioned in the chapter?

Exercise 5

Developing a Coding Framework for Data Analysis

Option A

Think about your own study and based on the research questions you have developed and your study design, create a draft coding framework. As you are putting it together, ask yourself the following questions:

1. What are the main codes that would be relevant to my research questions?
2. Based on the theoretical framework you have selected for your study, do you need to add any other potential codes?
3. Review your coding framework. What codes might be missing?

Option B

Think about the case study presented in Exercise 4. Based on the research questions you have developed and the study design, create a draft coding framework. As you are putting it together, ask yourself the following questions:

1. What are the main codes that would be relevant to my research questions?
2. Would you need to add any other potential codes depending on the theoretical framework you are using?
3. Review your coding framework. What codes might be missing?

Case study: Programme to support parents of children with learning disabilities

A new programme aimed at supporting parents of children with learning disabilities is being rolled out across three neighbourhoods through their local community centres. Your team has been asked to develop a rapid qualitative study with the aim of documenting the process of implementation and capture lessons learnt that could be used to inform the rollout of the programme in other neighbourhoods.

Your team is composed of three full-time researchers. The study should not last more than six months and emerging findings need to be shared two months after the study start date to inform decisions that need to be made during the early implementation phase.

6

CHALLENGES AND PRACTICALITIES OF RAPID QUALITATIVE RESEARCH

In Chapter 1, I briefly summarised some of the challenges of rapid qualitative research outlined in the literature. In this chapter, I dig a little deeper into these challenges, highlighting how these might manifest in practice, what we and other teams have done to address them and areas that we still need to work on to make sure we are able to carry out high-quality research in short amounts of time. I focus on four main types of challenges: challenges related to ethics and governance, team-work challenges, challenges related to rapid access and coverage, and those that might shape data quality (validity and credibility of the research).

Ethics and Governance

When we discuss streamlining study timelines with other research teams, a comment we hear frequently is that the world of ethical governance and research review is not prepared for rapid qualitative research. Delays produced by the review of studies by research ethics committees in universities as well as clinical settings have been frequently reported in the literature (Driscoll et al., 2008; Iedema et al., 2012; Polito et al., 2014). In addition, several scholars have argued that these review processes have been designed for the review of clinical trials and cannot always be adapted to the features and demands of qualitative research. In addition to these limitations, rapid qualitative research continues to be an uncommon type of research design, leading to misunderstanding between research teams and ethics committees and producing even more delays in approvals. Fast-track review processes have been produced in several countries, such as:

- Expedited review process for low-risk studies in the US Institutional Review Boards (IRBs)
- Proportionate review process for low-risk studies by the Health Research Authority (HRA) in England and Wales
- Review by Chair only (vs full ethics committee) for low-risk studies in university Research Ethics Committees (RECs) in UK universities

Despite these fast-track processes, ethical review continues to be a contributing factor to delays in the set-up of rapid studies and has even deterred teams from engaging in rapid qualitative research. During the COVID-19 pandemic, we developed a series of 'mirror studies' for a rapid appraisal on the experiences of frontline staff across 22 countries. We discussed the project with several teams who ultimately ended up deciding that they would not participate in this international collaborative project because local ethics committees would not be able to review and approve the study in a rapid way. They felt they would lose valuable data and did not have the resources, energy or interest in engaging in lengthy and cumbersome administrative processes.

The COVID-19 pandemic radically transformed the processes for the review of research studies in the United Kingdom and, for instance, our rapid appraisal was reviewed and approved in under two weeks. It was the first qualitative study on COVID-19 to be approved in the country and we were collecting data a few days after approval. As universities and hospitals are now beginning to transition back into their normal ways of working, a question that remains is the extent to which these rapid review processes could remain for studies on issues that are time-sensitive (beyond the topic of infectious epidemics) or that need to use a rapid research design (McNally, 2020).

In addition to the high-risk and low-risk review tracks outlined earlier, could an additional review process be established for rapid research? What would review criteria for this type of research look like and would the creation of this separate track produce more harm (by creating an additional layer of infrastructure required for review) than good? In a previous publication, I have analysed the processes used by ethical review board committees in organisations such as Médecins Sans Frontières that are used to the implementation of research on time-sensitive topics and contexts (Vindrola-Padros, 2020). An in-depth exploration of these processes as well as those established by countries around the world during the COVID-19 pandemic might be able to shed light on potential ways forward in the development of ethical review processes that are suitable for rapid qualitative research.

Team-Based Fieldwork and Analysis

One of the challenges of team-based rapid qualitative research identified in the literature is the integration of researchers in large teams who might not have extensive qualitative research experience (Bentley et al., 1988). The use of inexperienced researchers means that some time needs to be spent upskilling members of the team, which might delay study set-up and the start of data collection. It might also complicate or slowdown other stages of the research such as data analysis. These are challenges that can be present in any type of study, but there is little room for delays in rapid qualitative studies. As a response to this situation, some authors have developed strategies for intensive team training for local field researchers (i.e. community members tasked with the role of researchers for the first time) and junior researchers (i.e. team members who have formally trained as researcher, but might be participating in a study for the first time) or novices to rapid qualitative research (i.e. experienced qualitative researchers who do not have knowledge or experience of rapid qualitative research approaches).

Training

One of the most complete intensive training programmes for field researchers I have seen to date is the one developed for rapid assessment response and evaluation (RARE) by Brown et al. (2008). I have summarised this programme in Chapter 2 (Table 2.4). It involves three days of intensive training and covers the history of rapid qualitative research, the steps involved in carrying out interviews, focus groups and observations, and practical exercises involving carrying out observations and developing fieldnotes, designing an interview topic guide and developing a stakeholder group. Beebe (2001, 2014) has also developed a training programme on rapid assessment process and rapid qualitative inquiry (RQI) (see Table 6.1).

Table 6.1 Summary of a training programme for field researchers developed by Beebe (2001, 2014).

Orientation
• Introduction to qualitative research
• General overview of rapid qualitative inquiry (RQI)
Practice team interview and group analysis
• Teams of at least two people carry out a team interview of about ten minutes
• The team first practise putting together and piloting an interview topic guide
• After the interview, the team discuss the content and main learning from participating in the interview process
Mini-RAP
• Short research activity composed of: two interviews of at least 15 minutes (carried out by a team of at least two people), time to prepare interview questions, time in between interviews to discuss the content, and preparation of preliminary findings

Our team has also developed a series of one-day intensive training courses providing a general overview of rapid qualitative research as well as in-depth training on specific rapid approaches such as rapid evaluations and rapid ethnographies. We have organised the training based on five main features:

1 ***Practice-based:*** Learning while doing is more effective so the training in based on a series of practical exercises that involve the design and hypothetical implementation of rapid research.
2 ***Collaborative:*** The practical exercises mentioned earlier are carried out as part of a team to simulate research team discussions and decision-makings processes common to most rapid qualitative research.

3 ***Relevant:*** The training is continuously updated and relies on the use of current examples from the field of rapid qualitative research.
4 ***Participant-led:*** The content and format of delivery is adapted to suit the needs and interests of course participants. Opportunities are also generated for peer-to-peer learning, where the instructor mainly acts as a facilitator.
5 ***Intensive:*** Each course only requires one day for delivery so it can be easily integrated into rapid research timelines. All courses are designed to provide overviews of topics and act as a signposting exercise for deeper learning. Instructors provide lists of resources and refer to them throughout the course in case participants need to explore specific topics in greater depth after the course and while putting their new skills into practice during the implementation of their rapid studies.

Consistency across Team Members

One of the main challenges of any type of team-based research, whether rapid or not, is the need to maintain consistency in data collection and analysis across all researchers. In the case of rapid research, however, timelines might be compressed to the extent that common forms of cross-checking are not possible. As mentioned in Chapters 4 and 5, one of the ways in which some teams overcame this challenge was through the use of structured ways of collecting data, such as manuals or guides. These take different forms and have mainly relied on the use of tables or other types of pre-established forms to make sure all researchers collect data in the same way. In cases where an iterative design is applied and adaptation of these tools as the research is ongoing is allowed, constant communication is required between researchers to make sure any changes made to the forms are replicated across all researchers.

This structured approach has also been applied in the data analysis phase through the use of codebooks or pre-established coding frameworks (see Chapter 5) as these provide a detailed guide for researchers and seek to ensure consistency in coding across researchers. Despite these structured approaches, many researchers have opted for adding layers of cross-checking in the form of a member of the team who is assigned to this role (Bikker et al., 2017). 'Cross-checker roles' have been used in data collection and analysis and this person is responsible for going through the data as it is being collected or analysed, identifying inconsistencies and bringing these up for discussion during team meetings. It is then up to the team to agree how to address the inconsistencies in data collection or analysis generated so far and develop a strategy for moving forward where these can be reduced.

Team Reflexivity

We have sought to add another layer to the rapid research we carry out as a team. This can be thought of as a cross-checking exercise, but one that goes beyond stages of data collection and analysis in specific projects and critically analyses our working dynamics as a team. We have established a team reflexivity approach, where we continuously reflect on our positionality and practices as individual researchers, as part of a team and when interacting with external actors (including research participants, organisations, clients and other stakeholders). The aim of our team reflexivity is to reflect on these interactions, how they make us feel and think, and shape the way in which we produce, share and use knowledge. This approach involves critical scrutiny of our practices as a team on a continuous basis, always searching for ways in which we can improve how we design studies, train and support members of the team, liaise with clients and other stakeholders, collect and analyse data, use social theory, share findings, guarantee the use of findings, and contribute to wider discussions within the rapid qualitative research field (see Figure 6.1).

Many of these reflections are abstract and happen on an ad hoc basis, but, in order to ensure their continuity and make sure team reflexivity is firmly embedded in our ways of working, we have integrated it into our daily activity. A space for team-based reflection is built into all of our team meetings. These might happen monthly or more frequently if we are implementing very rapid studies (could be twice a week or weekly). We use this space to reflect on anything related to our practice as a team that should be discussed with others. This can include practical discussions in relation to not feeling supported or with the appropriate skills to carry out a particular task or more abstract discussions

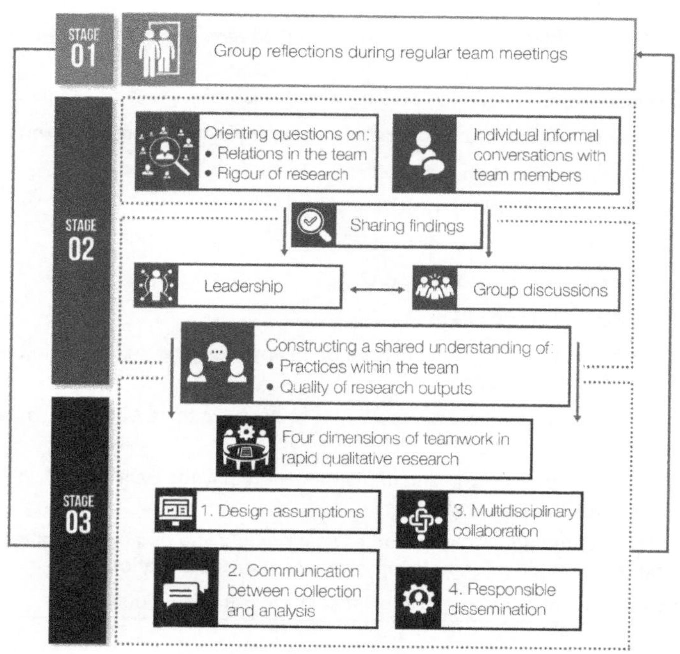

Figure 6.1 Team reflexive model (Source: Rankl et al., 2021)

about the future direction of the team and the extent to which we should be changing our areas of focus.

We have also developed a rapid qualitative study where we carried out interviews with members of our own team, frequent collaborators, previous clients and individuals who might have used our study findings. The interviews are normally conducted by new researchers or those who might be carrying out temporary placements to make sure there is some degree of external input into the process. We do this more formal process of data collection once a year. The last time we carried out these interviews, we used the interview topic guide included in Table 6.2.

Interviews were carried out via telephone or through video calls and were audio recorded. The researcher took notes during the interviews and used a rapid assessment procedures (RAP) sheet to summarise emerging findings. We maintained anonymity throughout data collection and analysis and once the main study findings were recorded on the RAP sheets, the audio recordings were deleted, so other members of the team could not have access to them. The researcher who carried out the interview shared the main findings with team leads and these were then discussed in depth during team

Table 6.2 Summary of the main questions used in the interview topic guide used to facilitate team reflexivity (Rankl et al., 2021)

What is the role you currently play within the team?
How did you join the team?
How long have you been working as part of the team?
Why did you join the team?
Would you like to have a different, or ongoing role with the team, beyond what you are doing now? Why or why not?
Can you describe your overall experience working with the team?
How has your experience with the team compared to your expectations when joining?
What are some of the things the team does well?
What are the areas that need to be improved?
Have you felt supported in your work by the team?
If yes, what was the most useful type of support?
If no, what type of support did you need?
If you worked/currently work with other teams, are there any tools/approaches from our team you would implement in these settings/projects?
When thinking about the studies implemented by the team, have there been any limitations in their design and implementation?
Are there any limitations in their design and implementation that you believe you would not or have not encountered in other long-term projects?
If we were to design and implement these studies again, would you do anything differently? Would you have any suggestions to offer for their improvement and/or adaptation?
Is there anything else you think we should know that I have not asked you today?

meetings. The findings were also shared before the team's annual strategy meeting and were incorporated into activities for the next academic year. The questions in the topic guide and the notes taken from the meeting minutes represent a starting point of more in-depth discussions in relation to the work we do, its impact and how we should work in the future (for a detailed description of this process, see Rankl et al., 2021).

The last time we carried out this exercise, it pointed to interesting and important dimensions in relation to our ways of working. There was a degree of mismatch between how the team leads, senior researchers and junior researchers visualised the team and the studies we were carrying out at that time. While the leads were aiming for the establishment of more distributed forms of leadership, where different members of the team could be given the opportunity to lead different streams of work, improving leadership skills and generating ownership over specific aspects of the work, senior researchers felt this model increased their responsibility over milestones and more junior members of the team (and this was seen as a burden). A reflection made by senior researchers on the team was that the rapid studies they were leading on required a balance in relation to experienced and inexperienced researchers to facilitate leadership in the context of time pressures. This finding prompted us to reflect on our internal team structure and consider additional approaches to governance and project management. After careful consideration, we decided to continue with a similar leadership approach as we felt that our distributed leadership and somewhat flat hierarchies were core components of our team philosophy, but decided to maintain clear communication across the team in relation to our perceived benefits of this model as well as expectations of the workstream lead role. We also looked carefully at the skills required across the team and developed an internal training programme to make sure junior researchers and new researchers joining the team were supported centrally (and removed this responsibility from the workstream leads).

In addition to questioning how we work, we have also used team reflexivity to explore the limitations of the knowledge we produce. The last time we carried out this exercise, common limitations of rapid qualitative research (i.e. 'snapshot lens', focused, too structured, etc.) were mentioned, but an interesting discussion emerged in relation to our study on the experiences and perceptions of healthcare workers (HCWs) during the COVID-19 pandemic in the United Kingdom (see case study in Chapter 8). Members of the team rightfully highlighted a major oversight in our study design in relation to capturing the points of view of HCWs from lower-ranking jobs (i.e. domestic staff, porters, healthcare assistants) and those from ethnic minority backgrounds.

When we designed the study, we were in pre-peak stages of the pandemic where we were focusing our attention on the impact of COVID-19 on staff working in the emergency department and intensive care units (ICUs). Even though we later adapted our sampling framework to capture the views of other HCWs playing a role in the response (i.e. physiotherapists, pharmacists, etc.), we did not move quickly enough to generate a diverse enough sample of study participants. This has meant that, even though we have attempted to analyse the data to capture a wide range of experiences, there will be an inextricable bias in our interpretation of the data due to a sample that does not reflect the ethnic and lower-ranking job composition of the National Health Service (NHS). Nonetheless, this experience has generated useful learning for future studies and our sampling framework design (in theory and practice), even in studies where we are incredibly pressed for time.

Relationships with Study Participants

Another frequently mentioned challenge in rapid qualitative research is that, due to the short duration of fieldwork, researchers are not able to generate the same type of in-depth relationships with study participants as in long-term research. Without discounting the fact that time in a specific setting might lead to the development of strong relationships with participants, in our experience, relationship-building has more to do with the predisposition of the researcher to build these relationships than with the amount of time spent in a particular place. As discussed in Chapter 3, relationship-building needs to be seen by the research team as a way of developing rapport with participants and considered a component of the process of generating data. Long-term presence is not enough (as we have countless examples of long studies where relationships were not developed) and rapid studies have integrated different strategies to develop relationships with research participants, even if the length of the face-to-face fieldwork is limited.

We have also experienced relationship-making as a dynamic process that might entail the following stages:

- ***Extending relationships from previous studies:*** Many of the rapid studies we have carried out are in settings where we have worked previously. Despite focusing on a different topic, we tend to interact with the same people and continue to build and reinforce existing relationships.
- ***Relationships outside of study data collection periods:*** We consider fieldwork to encompass time beyond active data collection as we are analysing data in greater depth, developing reports or other materials for dissemination. The reason for this wider representation of fieldwork is that we continue to collect and make sense of data during these stages, but we also continue to communicate with research participants. This communication might be established to provide an update in relation to the study, seek clarification in relation to collected data or be more informal and be used to check-in and see how people are doing. This communication might be face to face but is frequently enacted through email, phone or group chats.
- ***Intensive data collection:*** Some authors have argued that in-depth relationships can be created in short-term research as these studies might rely on more intensive forms of data collection, where the researcher spends longer periods of time per day in the field (increasing the intensity of contact with research participants) but the overall duration of the fieldwork is shorter. One example of this intensive design and how it differs from

long-term research can be the modification in shadowing we made for a recent rapid ethnography. When we normally shadow healthcare staff (i.e. follow them around as they carry out their routine daily activities to understand their movement through spaces, how they occupy their time, who they interact with, etc.) we organise shadowing sessions of two hours per day to reduce the burden on the healthcare staff and the exhaustion of the researcher. We might shadow one staff member one day and then come back and shadow the same staff member or a different one another day. When carrying out a rapid ethnography, this might need to be designed differently as we might not be able to come back for several days to complete the shadowing. This would mean that the researcher might need to shadow the member of staff for a longer period of time (with breaks in between), they might shadow two different staff members on the same day, or there might be two different members of the team shadowing different members of staff on the same day. We might need to consider shadowing on different days or at different times of day to capture potential changes. This might be organised in a targeted way to ensure it does not increase the duration of the data collection period or it might be combined with other data collection tasks that can be carried out in parallel. In other words, the length of the study might be shorter, but the hours of contact with individual participants might be more when compared to long studies.

Rigour

As explored in Chapter 1, one of the reasons why rapid qualitative research has a bad reputation is due to concerns about the robustness of study designs and the validity of the findings. We have spent a considerable amount of time examining rapid qualitative research designs and have reached the conclusion that the speed of the study is not related to its overall rigour. In other words, the issue is not the length of the study, but how it is designed and carried out. We have pointed to the areas of good practice for the design and implementation of rapid qualitative research throughout the book. Nonetheless, we still consider it important to engage in a discussion in relation to the quality of rapid studies and standards for their design and the reporting of findings.

In two reviews on the implementation of rapid research in healthcare sectors, we found gaps in reporting of study designs that made it impossible for us to assess the quality of the studies (Johnson and Vindrola-Padros, 2017; Vindrola-Padros and Vindrola-Padros, 2018). Some gaps in reporting were considerable, such as failing to describe the study sample or the methods used for data analysis. These findings led us to consider the importance of developing standards for rapid qualitative research that are different to existing standards for qualitative research (Vindrola-Padros, 2020). The notion of standards for qualitative research has been contested as several authors have argued that there is no consensus regarding the 'best' way to design and implement qualitative research and cautioned that the mainstream use of these standards could limit the options available for qualitative research design, reduce creativity and restrict the production of new knowledge (Freeman et al., 2007; Popay et al., 1998).

However, proponents of the use of standards have argued that these can improve the transparency and completeness of reporting and increase the quality of studies (Moher et al., 2010; Tong et al., 2007). Reporting standards can provide a framework for the review and assessment of studies and facilitate the use of findings. In our case, we think that the field of rapid qualitative research could benefit from standards that encourage researchers to clearly report the details of study design and implementation, not so much with the aim of establishing an external claim of quality in relation to these, but as a way to learn from their approaches. This would entail transparent reporting in relation to changes made in the design as the study was ongoing, reasons why these changes were made and how these decisions were negotiated within teams. The aim would be to gain insight into the factors that act as barriers in rapid qualitative research or generate pressures that researchers need to respond to and understand the strategies rapid research teams have used to address them.

The only attempt at developing standards I have come across are the 11 criteria for RAP developed by Utarini et al. (2001). These criteria cover a range of questions that researchers can use to design and report the findings from rapid studies such as:

- Is the aim of the study clearly described?
- Are the researchers' background, prior knowledge and relationship to the community and cultural competence clearly presented and addressed?
- Is there an adequate description of the field guide (i.e. document outlining the approaches used in fieldwork) and rationale and process of its development?
- Is the recruitment process and training of research assistants presented, and is it sound?
- Is the rationale for the data collection methods and types of information collected with each method clearly presented?
- Is an appropriate strategy for selecting the study area(s) or research site(s) described?
- Is a systematic process of selecting informants used and is it adequately described?
- Is a strategy for assessing the credibility of the researcher and the study established and presented?
- Is the analysis process adequately described and was it sound?
- Are the findings and discussion clearly presented?
- Are ethical principles respected and is the process for informed consent described? (Utarini et al. 2001).

I think these are a useful starting point for the development of standards that could also be suitable for other types of rapid research approaches. Several of these questions, however, can be applicable to any type of research design (not only rapid studies) and rely on the user's interpretation of 'sound recruitment strategies', assessment of credibility or adequate description of analysis processes. In Table 6.3, I have included some questions that I think would need to be added to those originally developed by Utarini et al. (2001). These could be used to generate discussion and reach consensus within the wider rapid qualitative research field in relation to the steps in the design and reporting that would need to be taken into consideration by rapid research teams.

Table 6.3 Questions that could be considered for the development of reporting standards for rapid qualitative research

Study rationale	Did the idea for the study emerge from the research team or was it requested/commissioned by another organisation/actor? Are the findings required to inform any decisions? Who were the key study stakeholders?
Aims	What are the research questions or the aims of the study and how have these been developed? Were these co-designed with external actors? If so, what were the processes used to co-design them? Did the authors describe the theoretical perspectives used to inform these questions?
Scoping	Did the team carry out any scoping to determine the research questions and design the study? If so, how was the scoping designed and implemented?
Research team and reflexivity	What is the composition, field and level of expertise with rapid qualitative research of the members of the research team? Does the team include any community members or other researchers who are 'insiders'? If inexperienced researchers have been included, how have they been trained? Have the authors reflected on their own positionality throughout the research? Did they employ any strategies for individual or team reflexivity?
Study protocol	Has the study protocol been described? Were any changes made in the protocol prior to the beginning of data collection? If so, why were these changes made?
Data collection	Were any rapid techniques for data collection used? If the study was team-based, did the authors use any strategies for the cross-checking of data collection? Were any changes made in the study design during data collection? If so, why were these changes made? How were decisions in relation to these changes made?
Sampling	Did the authors present the original sampling framework? Were any changes made, why were they made and how were decisions about changes in sampling made? Did the authors acknowledge any limitations in sampling generated by the rapid nature of the study? Did the authors acknowledge any issues accessing potential participants?
Data analysis	Were any rapid techniques for data analysis used? If the study was team-based, did the authors use any strategies for the cross-checking of data analysis? Did the authors use other cross-checking interpretation techniques such as member checking? Were any changes made in the study design during data analysis? If so, why were these changes made? How were decisions in relation to these changes made? Did the authors analyse and collect data in parallel? If so, what techniques did they use to facilitate this process?
Ethical considerations	Was the study reviewed by a research ethics committee? If not, did it undergo any review processes? If not, why not? Were review processes streamlined in any way (i.e. through expedited reviews or exemptions from full committee review)? Were ethical principles (confidentiality, anonymity, voluntary participation, informed consent, minimising harm) maintained? If the authors reported any problems with these principles, how were they addressed?

(Continued)

Table 6.3 (Continued)

Sharing of findings	How and with what frequency were study findings shared with relevant stakeholders? How was this format and frequency agreed? Were emerging findings shared as the study was ongoing?
Limitations	Have the authors identified the limitations of the study? Were these anticipated or were they unexpected? Did the authors do anything to try to address the limitations?
Study duration	What was the total duration of the study and how much time was spent for its different phases? Did the authors encounter any delays and what were the reasons for these delays? Did the authors need to request any study extensions?
Use of findings	Have the authors indicated if and how the findings from the study were used? If the findings were not used, did the authors indicate why? If they were used, were the findings used in the short term, long term or both?

Next steps in relation to these questions will be to formulate them into potential reporting standards, test their applicability and develop a detailed description of how they could be implemented in practice. It is important to remember that I am not seeking to generate an external measure of quality that could potentially limit the diversity of rapid qualitative research. On the contrary, I think that clear reporting can help invigorate the field of rapid qualitative research as we will be able to learn from each other to experiment and generate new approaches to research.

Funding

A frequent question I receive when teaching rapid qualitative researchers who have been working on these types of studies for a long time is how we are able to maintain the sustainability of our team. Teams working on rapid studies who obtain funding per project are often faced with the challenge of maintaining staff with relatively stable full-time contracts even if the funding they obtain is only for a few months. These teams have to creatively combine rapid with longer-term studies or might need to carry out multiple rapid studies at the same time to cover different percentages of part-time contracts for researchers.

More traditional ways of obtaining funding in academia through grants and similar types of awards might not be enough, although, in the United Kingdom two rapid service evaluation teams have obtained funding for five years through the National Institute for Health Research (NIHR) Health Service and Delivery Research (HS&DR) programme. More commonly, however, rapid qualitative research teams based in universities will need to rely on what we refer to as 'hybrid' models of funding, where the team continues to apply for grants to fund specific projects as well as bid for tenders that can be brought into the university in the form of consultancies.

Over the past year, our team has combined funding from six consultancies to fund different percentages of the salaries of four researchers (three senior researchers and a junior one). The projects were staggered to give funding continuity to the researchers on the team and we had to bring in an additional researcher to cover one of the projects as we had reached maximum capacity in relation to workload. The addition of a new, temporary, researcher was arranged quickly as, over the years, we have developed a pool of researchers with different types of expertise interested in working with our team on a part-time basis. These researchers are based at universities and carry out part-time private work, are employed in other sectors such as non-governmental organisations (NGOs) or charities or work as private consultants on a full-time basis. Having this pre-established pool of researchers allows us to quickly set up studies based on the expertise we need.

We have also considered our team to be a teaching team in the sense that we continuously integrate undergraduate and graduate students into projects to help develop their research skills. These students normally work with us as our team projects are used to develop theses or dissertations and we have also established a training placement programme for those students interested in obtaining research experience independently of a formal degree. Many of the training tools mentioned in the book have been developed in collaboration with these students and, although training and ongoing support take time, we see these as opportunities for developing research capacity in rapid qualitative research in future generations.

Another aspect of the funding of rapid qualitative research we have explored has been the reduction of our normal research costs. In addition to salaries for staff, one of our highest expenses is funding for the transcription of interview or focus group recordings. We looked at the strategies other research teams were using for transcription and saw that these included bypassing transcription altogether by taking notes or analysing data directly from audio recordings (Neal et al., 2015; Vindrola-Padros and Johnson, 2020). Other teams have opted for selected transcription, where certain fragments of the recording are transcribed to save time and money. We have done this for several studies, but still carry out research where we think it's important to have a full transcript of the conversation. We are currently using voice recognition and transcription software to carry out the transcription in-house. We have reviewed several articles that describe the use of voice recognition software for transcription and have identified the limitations of these approaches such as errors that then need to be corrected (not saving time) (Vindrola-Padros and Johnson, 2020). Regardless of these limitations, our recent use of voice recognition has been relatively successful and has allowed us to carry out rapid research on a limited budget.

Chapter Summary

- Ethical review and approval processes continue to generate delays for researchers seeking to set up studies quickly.
- Team-based fieldwork and analysis can be facilitated through the training of inexperienced researchers, the development of tools for cross-checking data collection and analysis, and the establishment of approaches for team reflexivity.
- Recent reviews on rapid qualitative research approaches have pointed to gaps in the reporting of study design, implementation and dissemination strategies. One potential way of addressing these gaps could be through the development and widespread use of standards for reporting and assessment of rapid qualitative research.
- The sustainability of rapid qualitative research teams requires the use of 'hybrid' funding models, use of pools of part-time researchers, active integration and training of student researchers, and the use of cost-effective research strategies.

Discussion Questions

1. In your opinion, what are the top three challenges of carrying out rapid qualitative research?
2. Can you identify one way in which each of these has been addressed in practice?
3. What are other challenges rapid qualitative researchers might face that have not been mentioned in this book?

Exercise 6

The Challenges of Rapid Qualitative Research

Option A

Go back to the potential challenges you identified for your study in Exercise 1. Based on what you know now, do you think you would encounter these same challenges in the study? If so, what are some of the strategies from this chapter that you could use to address them? If not, are there other challenges you think you might encounter?

Option B

Go back to the potential challenges you identified for the study in Exercise 1. Based on what you know now, do you think you would encounter these same challenges in the study? If so, what are some of the strategies from this chapter that you could use to address them? If not, are there other challenges you think you might encounter?

School leaders noticed an increase in the number of children transferring to the school from areas that were not in its normal catchment area. These 'travelling' children were identified as having lower levels of attainment than the other children at the school and a higher level of social care needs. In order to identify the needs of incoming children and adapt their learning plans accordingly, the school headteacher contacted your team to carry out a rapid study focused on documenting children's (and their families') needs and experiences.

The research team had four part-time researchers available with expertise in qualitative and quantitative research. The school was not sure about the quality of its routinely collected data. Findings were required within a two-month timeframe to inform decisions regarding the adaptation of learning plans, but the study could be longer and additional findings be shared at a later date.

7

DISSEMINATION AND THE USE OF FINDINGS

When thinking about dissemination, our team has found it helpful to identify the main dissemination goal and then work backwards to identify what we need to do as a team to achieve it. This chapter mirrors this way of thinking and starts with some of the most common dissemination goals we have established for rapid qualitative studies. It then works backwards to discuss how we were able to achieve them within short study timeframes. When I use the term 'dissemination' in this chapter, I use it to refer to any type of sharing of findings (including verbal communication, short memos or reports, presentations, articles, workshops, etc.). I follow the definition of dissemination, used by Wilson et al. (2010), as 'a planned process that involves consideration of target audiences and the settings in which research findings are to be received and, where appropriate, communicating and interacting with wider policy and health service audiences in ways that will facilitate research uptake in decision-making processes and practice'. We have also found that multipronged dissemination strategies, that is, those that involve different audiences and different formats, are effective in rapid qualitative research.

Dissemination Goals

When thinking about dissemination goals, we ask ourselves the following questions:

1. Are we only attempting to share knowledge/information?
2. Do we want to use dissemination to cross-check data, obtain feedback, gain insight and/or generate engagement?
3. How frequently do we need to share findings and in what format?
4. Are there key deadlines for the sharing of findings?
5. Who will use the findings?
6. How will they use them?
7. What are their preferences for the format?

Depending on the answers to these questions, we are normally able to tease out dissemination goals that might fall into the following categories:

- Inform specific decisions that need to happen at particular times: capture the factors that played a role in the day-to-day running of a service or intervention, the problems faced by staff or users and strategies they used to overcome these.
- Develop a shared understanding of a situation or a problem.
- Inform the development of a future programme or intervention: capture a snapshot of a situation or the different dimensions of a problem.
- Shape an organisation's strategy.
- Contribute to the generation of an evidence-base in relation to a particular topic.
- Inform the development of a long-term, more in-depth study.
- Inform changes in policies or the design of new policies.

It is important to consider that dissemination goals might change as the project is ongoing, but setting goals early and in conjunction with those who will use or benefit from the findings creates an initial framework that can shape data collection and analysis. In other words, the dissemination goals will determine whether data collection and analysis need to happen in parallel, when cross-checking and synthesis of emerging findings need to happen, how these findings need to be developed in relation to presentation and the types of meetings or other types of encounters that need to be integrated in the research timeline.

Dissemination Mechanisms

In previous studies, we have used the following dissemination mechanisms:

- Frequent (weekly or every two weeks) sharing of findings in an accessible format (tables or lists of bullet points)
- Monthly presentations at meetings with stakeholders
- Sharing of emerging findings halfway through a study in the form of an infographic or short report
- Sharing of findings at the end of a study in the form of a short report
- Sharing of findings at the end of a study in the form of an animation

Most of our studies have combined two or more of these. In a recent book on rapid ethnographies (Vindrola-Padros, 2020), I have listed all of the formats we have used to share findings:

- One-page memos developed for each week of fieldwork
- Tables summarising the key findings per site
- Recorded narratives of sites and main findings in the form of podcasts

- Animations with the main study findings (to make these accessible to a broad audience)
- Short reports (printed)
- Visual summaries, animations and infographics
- Manuals for staff
- PowerPoint presentations
- Posters
- Leaflets
- Reports uploaded to websites
- Articles published in academic journals
- Articles published in non-academic journals
- News articles or press releases
- Book chapters
- Books

When attempting to disseminate findings to a broad audience or even when trying to make them accessible and rapidly understood, we have increasingly relied on visual approaches. Our favourite approach is a one-page infographic that can summarise the main findings and communicate them in a simple way. We develop infographics to accompany final reports but also use them as 'working documents' in the sense that we use them to share emerging findings. This involves sharing emerging findings with our lead user or client as well as study participants. I have included an example of this type of infographic in Chapter 8. We have also used infographics to explain the design of a study we are carrying out. This helps to rapidly spread the message of ongoing research, what it entails and how we plan to use the findings. The infographic included in Figure 7.1 was developed with the aim of disseminating a study we carried out in the United Kingdom exploring the experiences of healthcare workers during the COVID-19 pandemic and its replication across several countries around the world. It was an easy way of letting other teams know about the research and seeing whether they wanted to replicate the study in their countries. We also used it to explain the study to potential participants and sent it to them at the same time that we sent the participant information sheet.

We have also developed a different form of an infographic that we have described as a visual abstract. The aim of this visual material is to disseminate the findings of a research article that has been published recently. As we are an academic research team based in a university, a central form of dissemination for us continues to be through the publication of articles in peer-reviewed journals. These articles tend to be read by a small and selective audience, limiting the impact of our research. We have developed visual abstracts as a way of making these findings accessible to an audience that can span the academic environment. We circulate the visual abstract via social media, email and post it on our website (with a link to the original article, in case anyone wants to read it). Figure 7.2 includes an example of a visual abstract we developed recently to share the findings of an article on the implementation of rapid qualitative research during the COVID-19 pandemic (Vindrola-Padros et al., 2020).

COVID-19
RAPID MEDIA ANALYSIS:
DECEMBER 2019-PRESENT
Rapid review of newspaper and magazine articles and social media published from December 2019-present.
TWITTER
NEWSPAPER
MAGAZINE
RAPID APPRAISAL
BASED ON TELEPHONE INTERVIEWS
AIM
CAPTURE STAFF PERCEPTIONS AND EXPERIENCES WITH COVID-19
Purposive sample of staff including primary care, emergency departments and intensive care units (ICUs).
RAPID POLICY REVIEW
Review of policies and government guidelines in relation to COVID-19 and comparison of policies across countries.
'MIRROR STUDIES'
POLAND
UK
SWITZERLAND
ITALY
SPAIN
UNITED STATES
MEXICO
TAIWAN
NIGERIA
PAKISTAN
INDIA
DEMOCRATIC REPUBLIC CONGO
BRAZIL
INDONESIA
CHILE
ARGENTINA
SOUTH AFRICA
AUSTRALIA
Data across all countries will be synthesized to inform global response efforts.
The studies are coordinated by the Rapid Research Appraisal and Evaluation Lab (RREAL):
For more information, please contact Dr Cecilia Vindrola: c.vindrola@ucl.ac.uk
RREAL

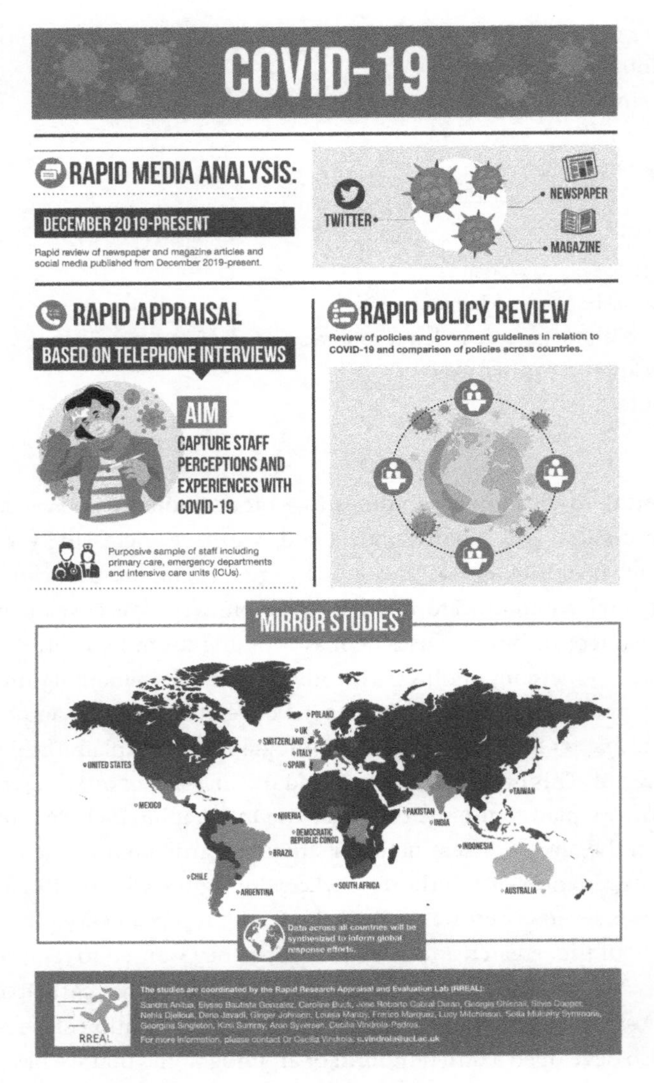

Figure 7.1 Infographic to advertise a COVID-19 study

Another visual material we have found useful for disseminating study findings to a broad audience is the use of animations. The animation is used to present the study design, information on the service, programme or area we are studying and the main findings. When working with organisations, in the public sector as well as non-governmental organisations, these animations have been well received as they can also be used by these organisations to showcase the work they have been doing. Recent examples of animations can be found on our website: www.rapidresearchandevaluation.com

CARRYING OUT RAPID QUALITATIVE RESEARCH DURING A PANDEMIC:
EMERGING LESSONS FROM COVID -19
RAPID RESEARCH
ETHICAL REVIEW
Some fast-track processes for ethical review have been established but these processes continue to delay the set-up of rapid studies.
COORDINATION
STANDARDS
More work needs to be done to establish standards of "good practice" to guide the implementation of rapid qualitative research.
RREAL

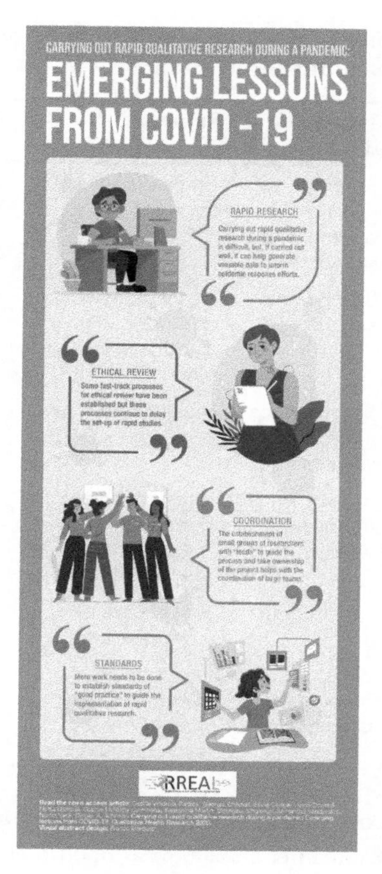

Figure 7.2 Visual abstract disseminating the findings presented in a research article

Dissemination Plans

The production of the outputs included earlier requires careful planning. After establishing the goals, we would then draft a detailed research timeline including stages of study set-up, collection and analysis and integrate different feedback loops or cycles based on the needs of our stakeholders. The benefit of a plan is that it allows us to think through the potential ways in which data can be interpreted, made sense of, visualised or presented and shared, even if it is in the form of interim findings as a team. Furthermore, developing a dissemination plan as a separate output to a study protocol enables us to have detailed discussions in relation to the sharing of findings with our key group of stakeholders. I have included an example of a dissemination plan in Table 7.1.

When developing the plan, we consider aspects of dissemination already identified in the literature such as dissemination goals, target audiences, key messages, sources/messengers,

Table 7.1 Dissemination plan for a rapid ethnography of a healthcare intervention (duration: six months)

Study stage	Time into study	Type of dissemination	Purpose	Format	Type of stakeholder
Scoping/ familiarisation	Week 1	Sharing research questions and study outline	Agree purpose of the study	Face-to-face meeting	Intervention designers, implementers and users
Scoping/ familiarisation	Week 2 or 3	Sharing final study scope	Final agreement on study design and dissemination plan	Email or face-to-face meeting	Intervention designers, implementers and users
Fieldwork and analysis	Month 2	Short memos (monthly or weekly)	Highlight emerging findings	Email	Implementers
Fieldwork and analysis	Months 3–4	Short memos (monthly or weekly)	Highlight emerging findings	Face to face	Intervention designers, implementers and users
Final analysis	Month 5	Report draft	Cross-check early interpretations	Email or face to face	Implementers
Writing	Month 6	Final report and presentation	Final sharing of findings and development of recommendations	Face to face	Intervention designers, implementers and users

dissemination activities, tools, timing and responsibilities, budget and evaluation of the impact of dissemination (Bauman et al., 2006; Zarinpoush et al., 2007). We extend these commonly used stages to question how we can adapt them to rapid qualitative research. We will ask ourselves, how can we produce high-quality and reliable findings in a limited study timeframe? How continuous should dissemination be? Who will have responsibility over the findings and their continuous dissemination? How can we share findings so they can be immediately actionable (easily translated into practice)? How can we reach a broad and diverse audience? How much of the funding can be used for dissemination? Who will be responsible for covering these costs? Can we think of cost-effective dissemination strategies?

This last point in relation to the budget is something we have thought a lot about. One strategy that has worked for us has been the integration of a graphic designer and other types of visual communicators as members of our research team. Our colleagues are allocated to a project like the researchers and they join team meetings, read study protocols and engage in conversations with stakeholders. Their contribution to these conversations means that the communication of study findings is thought about and discussed at all stages of the project. Their integration as part of the team also means that they are familiar with our vision and ways of working. Their role as team members enables them to inform the work of the team beyond individual projects and provide valuable input into the team strategy and long-term goals.

The implementation of a dissemination plan such as the one presented in Table 7.1 normally entails the design of feedback loops at specific times to share findings. Influenced by designs used in rapid evaluation (i.e. rapid feedback and rapid cycle evaluations), the concept of the feedback loop is based on the integration of an iterative perspective to research where data are collected, analysed, synthesised and shared on a continuous basis throughout the evaluation. The timing of the loops is decided with stakeholders and built into the dissemination plan. Loops might need to be eliminated or added throughout the study.

The establishment of feedback loops also allows us to obtain feedback from stakeholders on the study progress, the types of findings we are generating and other areas we might need to be focusing on. They function as a way of ratifying that the study is going according to their expectations and allow for any mid-study corrections we might need to consider. The sharing of findings early in the course of a study can also be used to secure engagement from stakeholders as they might be more interested in a study where they can get an idea of the type of output it will produce. This early engagement should not be underestimated as it might be required to secure access to people, areas or data necessary for the study. We examined the use of feedback loops in a recent review of rapid evaluations. I have presented these in Table 7.2.

Table 7.2 Examples of the steps involved in rapid feedback or rapid cycle evaluations

Rapid feedback evaluation (RFE)		**Rapid cycle evaluation (RCE)**	
Zakocs et al. (2015)	*McNall et al. (2004)*	*Schneeweiss et al. (2015)*	*Skillman et al. (2019)*
1. Clarify intent: Purpose, questions, study protocol	1. Collect existing data on programme performance	1. Review evaluation findings	1. Develop an analytic framework
2. Collect 'good enough' data: Collect and analyse data quickly	2. Collect new data on programme performance	2. Translate findings into actions	2. Collect data (first round)
3. Produce brief memo: Draft concise memo with main findings	3. Evaluate preliminary data	3. Make judgements based on findings	3. Analyse data and develop codebook
4. Engage in reflective debrief: Discuss findings with project team	4. Share findings/ recommendations with project team	4. Initiate implementation	4. Report findings
5. Decide whether more information is needed, take action or take no action	5. Develop and analyse alternative designs for full-scale evaluation	5. Make changes in implementation (if needed)	5. Collect data (second round) adding quantitative data
Repeat feedback loops (steps 2–5)	6. Assist in developing policy and management decisions		Repeat cycle (steps 3–5)

Source: Vindrola-Padros et al. (2021).

Multipronged Dissemination Strategies

Several rapid qualitative studies have implemented multipronged strategies for dissemination. For instance, Armstrong and Armstrong (2018) shared findings with the care homes where they conducted their research after one week of fieldwork, providing a list of 'promising practices' for the delivery of care. The research team gave presentations at the care homes after the study ended, held workshops, seminars and other events with relevant stakeholders (Armstrong and Armstrong, 2018). They also developed bookettes, that is, short and accessible paperback books with a summary of the findings. They were made available in multiple formats (print and online) and 'launched' at various public events (Baines and Gnanayutham, 2018).

When we make our dissemination plan, we consider the importance of combining multiple modes of dissemination to make sure the sharing of findings responds to different types of needs and preferences. The dissemination plan tends to cover different layers (including text-based and visually based formats, emerging and final findings, audiences that are specific and broad):

- Text-based sharing, normally in the form of one or multiple reports
- Brief and targeted visual sharing in the form of one or more infographics
- Longer and more in-depth visual sharing in the form of an animation or video
- Sharing allowing interaction and discussion in the form of presentations and/or workshops (producing slides or one to two summaries with tables or lists of bullet points)
- Sharing with an academic audience in the form of papers submitted to peer-reviewed journals (involving publishing study protocols, results from systematic reviews, research articles and articles where we discuss methodologies or the process of carrying out research)
- Sharing with a broader audience online and in text-based formats such as blogs or brief notes posted on our website
- Disseminating these outputs as well as additional ones via social media

Chapter Summary

- The identification of dissemination goals at the stage of study design can help inform the implementation of the data collection and analysis stages of the study.
- Dissemination plans can be used to establish clear deadlines by which emerging findings might need to be shared, the best format and audience, and the purpose of the dissemination.
- Dissemination plans should be agreed with all relevant stakeholders prior to the start of the study.
- Multipronged dissemination strategies are an effective way to ensure findings are shared to suit different needs and preferences.

Discussion Questions

1. What are the main components of a dissemination plan?
2. What are the different layers or dimensions of dissemination we attempt to cover in multipronged dissemination strategies?
3. What are additional dissemination strategies not discussed in the chapter?

Exercise 7

The Dissemination Plan

Option A

Based on the steps outlined in the chapter, identify the dissemination goals for your study and put together a draft dissemination plan (you can go back to the one you developed in Exercise 3 and revise it based on what you have learned so far).

Option B

Based on the steps outlined in the chapter, identify the dissemination goals for the case study from Exercise 3 and put together a draft dissemination plan.

Case study: Programme to support parents of children with learning disabilities

A new programme aimed at supporting parents of children with learning disabilities is being rolled out across three neighbourhoods through their local community centres. Your team has been asked to develop a rapid qualitative study with the aim of documenting the process of implementation and capture lessons learnt that could be used to inform the rollout of the programme in other neighbourhoods.

Your team is composed of three full-time researchers. The study should not last more than six months and emerging findings need to be shared in two months to inform decisions that need to be made during the early implementation phase.

8

CASE STUDY 1: A RAPID APPRAISAL OF HEALTHCARE WORKERS' EXPERIENCES OF CARE DURING COVID-19

The purpose of this chapter is to present the steps and challenges involved in the design and implementation of a rapid qualitative study in the context of a global pandemic, discussing the changes made due to pressures experienced in the field, unanticipated issues that emerged from the data, and the strategies the team implemented to maintain a clear focus to generate and share findings in a timely way. I present the rationale for the study, the original design and the different phases of implementation. I also discuss the changes made along the way, discussions we had as a team and the processes we used to make decisions in relation to these changes.

Rationale for the Study

Research on the design and implementation of epidemic response efforts at a global scale has pointed to the importance of considering staff perceptions and experiences of care delivery. Research from high-income settings has highlighted a series of factors that influence the behaviour of health workers during epidemics: fear of contagion, concern for family health, interpersonal isolation, quarantine, trust in and support from their organisation, information about risks and what is expected of them, and stigma (Ives et al., 2009; Koh et al., 2011; Maunder et al., 2010). Staff benefit from supportive supervision, peer support networks and good use of communication technology (Raven et al., 2018). Potential mitigating strategies included organisational implementation of infection prevention control (IPC) measures and complying with personal protective equipment (PPE) (Koh et al., 2011). All of these studies have called for more research into factors that influence healthcare workers' decisions to provide care at the frontline.

The COVID-19 outbreak that began in China in December 2019 set an unprecedented demand on healthcare systems across the world. There is evidence in global media that care delivery to critically ill patients has placed a burden on healthcare staff. Therefore, the concerns, intentions and behaviours of healthcare workers (HCWs) represent an important area of research (Michie, 2020). This rapid appraisal explored HCWs' perceptions and experiences of responding to the COVID-19 epidemic in the United Kingdom (Vindrola-Padros et al., 2020a).

Preparatory Work

We drew from our experience of carrying out rapid qualitative research in previous epidemics to identify key literature that we could use to inform our research questions and study design. We engaged early with key organisations informing epidemic response efforts in the United Kingdom. We also engaged with individual clinicians who would be delivering care on the frontlines to explore their ideas in relation to our study aims, how we should design the sampling and how study findings should be used. We liaised with other teams in the United Kingdom and abroad who were implementing or planning to implement similar studies. These discussions were helpful for identifying problems that were common across countries and to learn from the strategies implemented by other teams. These early discussions led to the creation of a global network of teams working on similar studies that communicated regularly.

Aims and Objectives

1. Explore the perceptions of HCWs in relation to COVID-19, and infected and potentially infected patients.
2. Explore the perceptions of HCWs in relation to the suitability of care delivery models and infrastructure to deal with the epidemic.
3. Identify the factors that shape clinical decision-making and action.

Research Questions

1. What are healthcare workers' (HCWs') perceptions of COVID-19, infected patients and potentially infected patients?
2. What are their experiences of delivering care in the context of this epidemic?
3. Do they feel like they have the proper training and supplies to work with patients potentially affected by COVID-19? If not, what additional resources would help them – both mentally and physically – do their work more effectively?

4 Do HCWs experience any concerns delivering care in this context? What are the underlying causes of these concerns with regard to the new virus and how can we address those concerns?

Design

In this study, we used a qualitative rapid appraisal design. Rapid appraisals were developed to collect and analyse data in a targeted way within limited timeframes and 'diagnose' a situation (Green and Thorogood, 2013). A rapid appraisal design often combines two or more methods of data collection and then uses triangulation from different sources as a form of data validation (Harris et al., 1997). It is based on an iterative process of collection and analysis, where 'the researchers begin with information collected in advance, and then progressively learn from each other and from information provided by semi-structured interviews and direct observations' (Beebe, 1995: 48). Based on our previous experience of carrying out research during previous epidemics and our knowledge of the literature on the implementation of rapid qualitative research in the context of complex health emergencies (Johnson and Vindrola-Padros, 2017), we selected a rapid appraisal design as it would allow us to:

- Make adaptations in the study design as the study was ongoing
- Implement strategies for team-based data collection and analysis, thus covering more ground in a shorter amount of time
- Carry out data collection and analysis in parallel, saving time, but also identifying emerging findings that could be shared in real time to inform epidemic response efforts

In the case of this study, we combined interviews with frontline staff with a rapid policy review and rapid media analysis.

Data Collection

Interviews

The study was based on telephone interviews with NHS staff. Semi-structured interviews were conducted via telephone with 60 healthcare workers. The interviews focused on perceptions of the virus, patients and the healthcare system.

Sampling

A purposive sample of 60 healthcare workers were selected for interview based on their role (see Table 8.1 for original sampling framework). The sampling strategy was informed by early preparatory work where we rapidly reviewed studies on epidemics with similar impact on the respiratory conditions of patients to identify the HCWs that would be more heavily impacted. We then had a few conversations with clinicians in acute care hospitals where we had worked before and where we hoped to base the study and asked for their feedback on our proposed sampling framework.

Table 8.1 Original sampling framework for healthcare worker interviews

Interviewee role/Professional group	Sector	Number of interviews
Emergency department consultants	Tertiary care (max. 3 Trusts)	10
Emergency department nursing staff	Tertiary care (max. 3 Trusts)	10
Emergency department management staff	Tertiary care (max. 3 Trusts)	5
Infection control staff	Tertiary care (max. 3 Trusts)	10
Microbiologists	Tertiary care (max. 3 Trusts)	5
Consultants in intensive care units (ICUs)	Tertiary care (max. 3 Trusts)	10
Nursing staff in ICUs	Tertiary care (max. 3 Trusts)	10
Overall total		60

Recruitment

Clinical leads approached staff to let them know about the study and make sure they were happy to be contacted by the research team. Staff members were then approached by the researcher via email and provided with a copy of the information sheet, which included details about the purpose, design, expectations, risks and benefits of the study. Staff were given 48 hours to decide if they would like to take part in the study. Staff who decided to take part in the study were asked to sign and email the researcher a consent form. The researcher proceeded to arrange a telephone interview at a time that was convenient for them.

Data Analysis

The analysis explored the most frequent topics originating from the interviews in relation to the research questions guiding this study. The data were analysed using framework analysis (Gale et al., 2013; Smith and Firth, 2011).

Rapid Policy Review

The aim of the review of healthcare policies was to understand how healthcare delivery had been reorganised in light of the COVID-19 pandemic.

The policy review was used to answer the main research questions guiding the study, but we also developed specific questions in relation to the policies:

1. What is the impact of COVID-19 on regular processes of healthcare delivery? (including care for COVID-19 positive patients and non-COVID-19 services)
2. Do policies vary by healthcare sector and/or patient groups?
3. Do policies change through time? Is it possible to identify the reasons why these policies change?
4. What are the policies being implemented to address the long-term effects of COVID-19 on healthcare systems?

Methods (Collection, Extraction and Analysis)

We carried out a rapid policy review based on the framework set out by Tricco et al. (2017) for rapid evidence synthesis. We searched for government policies in the United Kingdom published on the legislation.gov.uk and gov.uk databases using the terms: COVID-19 OR coronavirus OR corona. The search dates originally included 1 December 2019 to 8 June 2020 and have been updated on a weekly basis.

Inclusion criteria for the policies were:

- Published within the timeframe set out above
- Aimed at healthcare delivery
- Related to the COVID-19 pandemic

One reviewer selected the policies that met these criteria. A second reviewer extracted data based on pre-established categories and inputted the data on a spreadsheet. Data were cross-checked across reviewers. A third reviewer (with expertise in health systems analysis) identified the main topics emerging from the data and organised them into a conceptual framework. The framework became a working document that was modified as new policies were added to the analysis.

Rapid Media Analysis

We conducted a rapid media analysis of HCWs' perceptions and experiences with COVID-19 using the rapid evidence review method proposed by Tricco et al. (2017). The rapid review method follows a systematic review approach, but proposes adaptations to some of the steps to reduce the amount of time required to carry out the review (i.e. the use of large teams to review abstracts and full texts, and extract data; in lieu of dual screening and selection, a percentage of excluded articles is reviewed by a second reviewer, and software is used for data extraction and synthesis, as appropriate (Tricco et al., 2017)).

Even though this is a rapid media analysis, we used the Preferred Reporting Items for Systematic Reviews and Meta-Analysis (PRISMA) statement (Moher et al., 2009) to guide the reporting of the methods and findings.

Search Strategy

We conducted a review of published newspaper and magazine articles by running a search on the Nexis database. Results were exported in Excel spreadsheets. We also hand-searched other relevant newspaper and magazine articles in relevant media sources.

Selection

Following the rapid evidence review methodology (Tricco et al., 2017), one researcher screened the articles in the title and full text phases, and two researchers cross-checked exclusions. Disagreements were discussed until consensus was reached. The inclusion criteria used for study selection were:

- Focus on the perspectives or experiences of HCWs (self-reported or narrated in third person)
- Focus on the response strategies aimed at COVID-19
- Published from 1 December 2019 to 8 June 2020 and
- Published in English

Data Extraction and Management

The included articles were analysed using a data extraction form developed in REDCap (Research Electronic Data Capture). The form was developed after the initial screening of full-text articles. It was then piloted independently by two researchers using a random sample of five articles. Disagreements were discussed until consensus was reached. The data extraction form was finalised based on the findings from the pilot.

Data Synthesis

Data were exported from REDCap and the main article characteristics were synthesised. The information entered in free text boxes was exported from REDCap and analysed using framework analysis (Gale et al., 2013).

Ethical Review

The study was reviewed and approved by the Health Research Authority (HRA) in England and Wales (IRAS: 282069), and approved by local research offices of the hospitals where the study took place. Due to a fast-track review process established by the HRA, the study was reviewed and approved in seven days.

Research Team

The team began with three part-time researchers not directly funded for this study, but with some capacity to contribute to the study as their studies had been put on hold due to COVID-19. All non-essential studies or studies not linked to COVID-19 were put on hold in the United Kingdom until a few weeks after the epidemiological peak passed.

Original Study Timeline

The study was designed as a 12-month study to be able to capture changes in the pandemic over time, but data collection was front-loaded during the first months to capture perceptions pre-epidemiological peak, during the peak and post-epidemiological peak. This meant carrying out as many of the interviews as possible over a two-month period. We then had the option of adding another wave of interviews later in the year to capture the post-pandemic stages or experiences during a second or third surge in cases.

Budget

We did not have any funding in the form of grants available for this study. Due to the quick set-up of our study, there were no COVID-19-specific funding options available when we began data collection. As some of these options emerged, we were able to submit applications, but were unsuccessful. Nonetheless, we continued with the study using some of the options for saving on research costs outlined in Chapter 6 (transcribing in-house, using selected transcription). One of the reasons why we were able to carry out the study without a large budget was due to the freed capacity of some members of the research team. This was a unique situation produced by the pandemic. One of the reflections from our team in relation to external funding was the burden these applications generated for team leads who were already working longer hours than usual. There was a high rate of competition for these COVID-19-specific funding calls and the amount of work required to submit additional applications did not outweigh the benefits. Therefore, we decided to continue our study with our limited budget.

Study Life-Cycle: Month 1 (From Ethical Approval)

As mentioned above, we had originally planned to include HCWs from a maximum of three acute care hospitals and had sampled HCWs we knew would be more heavily affected by the pressures created by COVID-19. At the time of the study design, we were seeing that the most affected areas included emergency departments and intensive care units (ICUs). As we began data collection, however, we started to see that these groups tended to be relatively well protected in relation to PPE (at least in the hospitals where we were working), but other groups such as domestic staff and porters were not identified as high-risk, leading to some of the highest nosocomial infection rates in these professional groups. Many members of staff from these groups died in the United Kingdom. We decided it was important to submit an amendment for our original ethical review application to be able to include these professional groups as part of our sample. Reflections from our team through our team reflexivity exercises highlighted this as a major oversight in our study design, and, even though we made this amendment in the study design, we still had a considerable gap in our sample.

In this amendment, we also added another study site, which was a community care hospital. This meant that it was not a specialist hospital like our other sites and did not treat high-risk patients. Nevertheless, as data collection began, these types of hospitals began to play a bigger role delivering care for patients who did not need to be admitted into ICUs, but still needed to be hospitalised. There were also reports around the country that these types of hospitals had fewer resources in the form of PPE, well-being support for staff and training opportunities.

Our team suffered a notable expansion during this month, from the three researchers mentioned earlier, to an additional five researchers working on a part-time basis who volunteered their time as they wanted to make contributions to research informing response efforts. Most of these researchers were junior and this was their first experience with a qualitative study. This meant that they required considerable support from the team leads and senior researchers of the team before they could get started. We developed a step-by-step guide for interviewing for new members and established weekly team meetings to make sure they had plenty of opportunities to ask questions. Looking back, I think we should have tried to establish more formal training for new members (as we normally do in all of our studies), but the pressures generated by the pandemic (at home and at work) meant we did not consider this until it was too late.

As mentioned earlier, we engaged with a few organisations in charge of informing response efforts in the United Kingdom as we were designing the study. This meant that we were in close contact with them as data collection began. We were asked to deliver emerging findings in relation to HCWs' experiences that could be used to guide discussions and strategies in local hospitals on a regular basis, and during the peak, we were doing this twice a week. This frequent sharing of findings meant our team needed to be well coordinated, not only to cover a large volume of interviews per week, but also to analyse these and present key findings that the team lead could transform to an accessible format and share with these stakeholders. The processes outlined in Chapters 4 and 5 based on the use of RAP sheets facilitated this rapid sharing of emerging findings. Findings were shared in the form of tables or a list of bullet points and this synthesised approach was valued by these organisations (no one had time to read long reports).

During this month, we also developed a short commentary on the impact COVID-19 would have on Low- and Middle-Income Countries (LMICs). This was first submitted to a journal where the review process was too long, so we decided to remove the paper. We submitted to a different journal, but the review process took over four months, which meant that the piece was dated by the time it was reviewed. This experience made us reconsider the traditional publication route for studies in the future, including the publication of preprints before the submission of manuscripts to peer-reviewed journals.

Month 2

As the pandemic continued to evolve in the United Kingdom, we passed the peak but started engaging in conversations with HCWs in relation to the needs of patients who were discharged from ICU into other areas of the hospital and were eventually allowed to go home. HCWs were seeing that the virus was generating long-term effects, not only on patients admitted to hospital, but also those who seemed to be well enough to recover at home. Despite presumably few and low-risk symptoms, many of these patients were experiencing fatigue weeks after first experiencing symptoms. We started hearing about the impact of the virus on other organs beyond the respiratory track, generating renal failure, loss of cognitive function and motor coordination and heart failure. We started seeing how discussions in senior epidemic strategy groups (where one of our team leads acted as an expert in qualitative research) were including aspects of recovery and long-term rehabilitation that had not been mentioned previously.

Through our policy review, we also started capturing and analysing national policies and guidelines developed by professional organisations of physiotherapists, dieticians, and speech and language therapists aimed at alerting HCWs of the potential effects of ICU admission and the virus on motor coordination and the normal bodily functions of recovering COVID-19 patients. This led us to make a second change in our sampling strategy to include allied health professionals (physiotherapists, pharmacists, speech and language therapists, etc.). It also led to the expansion of our interview topic guide to include questions on recovery. At this time, a researcher joined the team with the interest of using the data to carry out a dissertation on the delivery of rehabilitation care to COVID-19 patients. She was also given the opportunity to move this workstream forward.

In addition to this graduate student, four others joined the team around this time. This expansion of the team coincided with our analysis of the data obtained to date to identify the areas of focus moving forward. As mentioned earlier, the initial stages of the study had a broad focus, documenting the experiences of HCWs without limiting these to particular topics. Our analysis of emerging findings allowed us to identify some of the key topics or concerns highlighted by HCWs (see Table 8.2). The new graduate students selected one of these topics for their dissertation and additional members of the team (core team members as well as volunteers) selected the remaining ones. We developed a system where one person acted as a 'team lead' and coordinated the analysis of data from the interviews, policy review and media analyses in relation to the area of focus. Everyone had the opportunity to sign up as a contributor to the different areas of focus depending on their interests and time availability. The team lead then coordinated the group by arranging frequent meetings to plan the analysis, discuss the emerging findings, develop the analytical framework, code the data, develop the themes and select the data that would be included in a paper for publication (see Figure 8.1 for a diagram describing the organisation of the team).

Table 8.2 Key areas of focus identified in month 2 of the study based on the concerns expressed by HCWs

Area of focus	Description
Emerging findings	General description of emerging findings based on data collected until the end of April 2020.
Well-being and mental health	Analysis exploring the mental health of frontline staff (current issues and potential long-term problems).
Emotions	An analysis of interview and social media data in relation to experiences of caring in the context of COVID-19.
Impact on the cancellation of elective surgery	Staff perceptions of the effects of COVID-19 on the cancellation of elective surgery and the long-term effects on patient care.
Personal protective equipment (PPE)	Explores the fears and concerns of HCWs about supply and adequacy, how workspaces are reorganised to manage infection, and how PPE influences patient care.
Patient recovery and rehabilitation	The experiences of HCWs delivering care to COVID-19 survivors dealing with respiratory issues, cognitive decline and muscle degeneration.
Staff redeployment	Uses the lens of resource scarcity to examine staff redeployment during the pandemic.
Care at end of life and palliative care	COVID-19 has changed staff experiences of working with dying patients and their families. While clinical care continues to be delivered, the large number of rapid deaths teamed with strict infection control measures, has led to an impact on healthcare workers' (HCWs) ability to provide compassionate care to patients.
Gender	Focus on how gender shapes care workers' experiences at hospital and at home.
BAME inequalities	BAME HCWs' experiences during the COVID-19 epidemic in the United Kingdom.

This identification of areas of focus led to another round of changes in the interview topic guide. The leads for the different areas met to review the existing topic guide and make decisions in relation to what could be removed and what needed to be added so the data required for each analysis was available. The revised topic guide was piloted and additional refinements were made. Each lead cross-checked the data in the RAP sheets and interview transcripts to make sure the data required for their individual analysis was available.

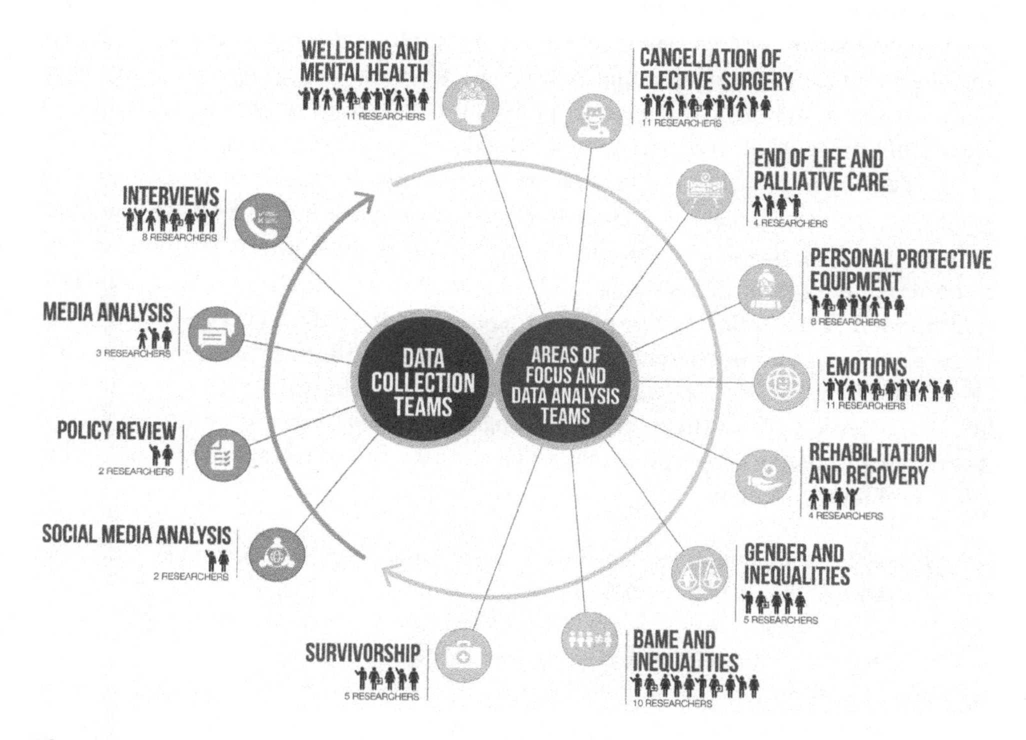

Figure 8.1 RREAL organisation across data collection and data analysis workstreams

Month 3

This month was characterised by a continuation of data collection across all data sources and analytical work that was happening in parallel. As we passed the epidemiological peak, the pressure to deliver findings with our partner organisations reduced and we were only sharing these on a fortnightly basis at this stage. This allowed the team to focus more in-depth on the analyses of data and start developing some manuscripts for publication. Two manuscripts were written up in parallel at this stage: (1) an emerging findings paper (Vindrola-Padros et al., 2020a) and (2) a methods paper focused on sharing our experience of designing and setting up rapid qualitative research during a pandemic (Vindrola-Padros et al., 2020b). Members of the team were asked if they wanted to contribute to the development of these manuscripts and I led the writing in both cases.

The first manuscript included everyone who had been involved in the study up to this date and the emerging findings included data from 30 interviews, 35 policies, 146,000 social media posts and 101 newspaper articles. The second manuscript included contributions from the members of the team who were interested in the methodological aspect of rapid qualitative research (self-identified) and included a reflection on designing, submitting for ethical review and setting up three studies during COVID-19 (the study I have been discussing on HCWs' experiences, a mixed-methods study on the use of qualitative data to inform epidemic response efforts and a global survey on the impact of COVID-19 on the delivery of cancer care). Due to an ever-expanding team and the development of multiple papers in parallel, we decided to propose clear guidelines in relation to authorship at this stage to manage expectations. Many of the researchers on the team had volunteered their time and, although they had done this in an altruistic way to make a contribution to epidemic response efforts, there were high expectations in relation to the number of publications where they could be named as authors. As in previous studies, we decided to follow the ICJME guidelines on authorship due to their clarity and the fact that we believed they set the right level of engagement of co-authors in the manuscript development process. These guidelines establish that manuscript authors are those that meet the following criteria:

- Substantial contributions to the conception or design of the work; or the acquisition, analysis, or interpretation of data for the work; AND
- Drafting the work or revising it critically for important intellectual content; AND
- Final approval of the version to be published; AND
- Agreement to be accountable for all aspects of the work in ensuring that questions related to the accuracy or integrity of any part of the work are appropriately investigated and resolved (ICJME, 2021).

The communication of these criteria for authorship was contentious as several team members were worried that this would mean that they would not be considered as authors for papers, even though they had spent considerable time collecting data. The team leads appeased these concerns by indicating that those who had collected data would be given the opportunity to take part in the analyses and contribute to the drafting of manuscripts. This was arranged through a document developed by one of the leads, where all areas of focus, leads and people contributing to the analyses were listed. Regardless of the approaches aimed at generating transparency, authorship continued to be a contentious issue throughout the study and an area we think we need to improve for future studies.

Team meetings continued with the same frequency (weekly for data collection teams) and fortnightly for full team meetings. We integrated the areas of focus into the agenda and used these meetings to review progress across all areas. We decided as a team that the next area of focus that needed to be prioritised was the work we wanted to carry out on the mental health and well-being of HCWs. A new researcher had joined our team who was a specialist in mental health and she suggested carrying out a quick analysis with the dataset that was complete up to that date (33 interviews) focusing on HCWs' experiences with the well-being support delivered in their hospitals. She also suggested carrying out a longer piece of work on HCWs' mental health in a few months, when we would have a complete dataset (130 interviews and complete policy and media reviews).

The analysis and write-up for the first paper on well-being was carried out in six weeks and involved 11 members of the team. It was an intensive process that entailed an analysis of interview data as well as a review of well-being guidelines published in the United Kingdom that was carried out in parallel and led by a researcher external to the team (with mental health expertise) who collaborated with us on this aspect of the work (San Juan et al., 2021). This paper was rejected by the first two journals where we submitted. We were encountering delays in the review process similar to those described for other papers, so before submitting to the third journal, we decided to publish the manuscript as a preprint (www.medrxiv.org/content/10.1101/2020.07.21.20156711v1).

Month 4

By this stage, we were seeing that new data in the media analysis on HCWs' experiences were limited. We decided to finish the regular searches of newspaper articles and social media we had been carrying out up to that time. We also decided to stop the regular searches with the policy review as the production of new policies and guidelines was reduced significantly after the first epidemiological peak. The interviews had also progressed significantly and we had reached our target at two hospitals. We continued working in a third hospital, but this required a smaller interview team. This meant we now had complete (or nearly complete in relation to the interviews) data sets where we could do more in-depth work.

Up to this date, the leads of the different areas of focus had been planning the analyses, but during this month, several teams began to develop analytical frameworks to bring together all streams of work and code the data (with the exception of the three papers mentioned before that were submitted for publication before this date). The team focusing on the impact of COVID-19 on the cancellation of elective surgery was the next one to move forward with their analysis (Singleton et al., 2021 under review). This team brought together findings from the policy review and developed a timeline on how the delivery of elective surgical procedures had changed in the United Kingdom during the different stages of the pandemic. It also combined social media data. Eleven members from the team participated in this paper. The analysis was led by a junior researcher who was supported by several senior researchers on the team. This team also had input from a researcher who could provide clinical input, an anaesthetist who joined the team due to her interest in qualitative research.

The team focusing on end-of-life and palliative care during COVID-19 was much smaller (only four members of the team) and this was due to limited interest in this topic. The analysis was led by a graduate student whose doctoral thesis was being developed in the field of palliative care (Mitchinson et al., 2021). She was also based in a palliative care department at the time. Three social scientists joined the team (one junior and two seniors) from psychology, sociology and anthropology, generating an interesting combination of expertise and perspectives.

Month 5

When we reached this month, we had already carried out 114 interviews with HCWs (surpassing the 60 set out in the original protocol). We felt it was the right time to share emerging findings with those who had shared their stories with us. All area leads were asked to develop a couple of lines on the key high-level findings coming out of their analyses. These were then discussed at a team meeting with our graphic designer and he developed the infographic in Figure 8.2 as a way to share emerging findings with the HCWs who took part in the study, across hospitals and with other relevant organisations.

When sent out to the HCWs who took part in the interviews, this early sharing of findings was also used as a member checking exercise, where we asked participants to provide feedback on our interpretation of the findings. This feedback was incorporated into our final analysis of the findings across the different areas of work.

Our methodological paper on the lessons learnt while carrying out rapid qualitative research during the COVID-19 pandemic was published during this month (Vindrola-Padros et al., 2020). In order to increase its accessibility, we developed the visual abstract presented in Chapter 7 (Figure 7.2), in collaboration with our team's graphic designer.

This month was characterised by the wrapping up of the four analyses that were developed as part of graduate theses. These included theses and subsequent papers on: HCWs' experiences with PPE (Hoernke et al., 2021 and Figure 8.3), HCWs' perspectives on delivering rehabilitation care for recovered COVID-19 patients and the future delivery of this care (Lewis-Jackson et al., under review), and gender inequalities in the experiences of HCWs during the pandemic (Regenold & Vindrola-Padros, 2021).

Another group within the team, composed of 11 members, began to work on another workstream focused on integrating theoretical perspectives on caring and care work into an analysis of the emotional labour involved in HCWs' experiences of delivering care during the pandemic (Dowrick et al., under review). This analysis followed the same steps as those used in the well-being paper and the one that focused on the cancellation of elective surgery. Team members contributed expertise in medical anthropology, sociology, psychology and public health.

Month 6

As I was putting together this book manuscript, we were beginning with the work for this month of the study, which marked significant changes in relation to the composition of our team. The researchers who had joined the team on a voluntary basis now had to return

COVID-19

RAPID MEDIA ANALYSIS:

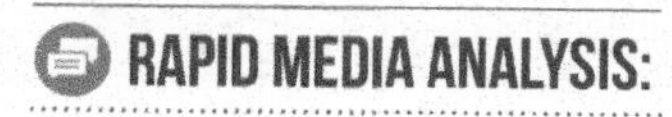

Rapid review of 150 newspaper articles and 146,000 social media posts from December 2019 to June 2020.

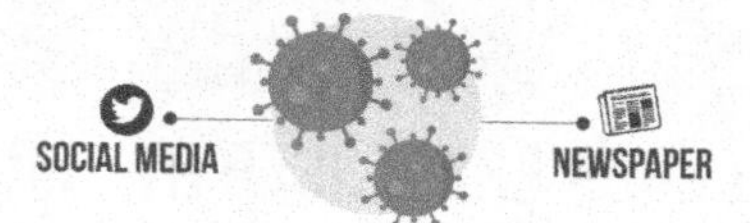

TELEPHONE INTERVIEWS WITH FRONTLINE WORKERS

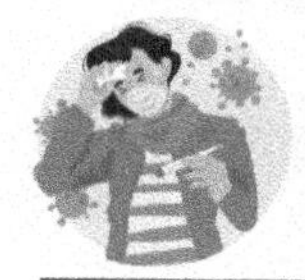

Purposive sample of 130 workers delivering care on the frontline to capture their experiences during the pandemic.

RAPID POLICY REVIEW

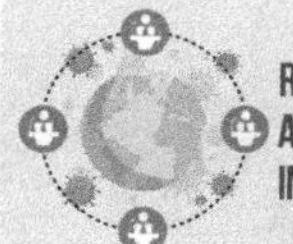

REVIEW OF 70 UK POLICIES AND GOVERNMENT GUIDELINES IN RELATION TO COVID-19.

COVID-19 EMERGING FINDINGS

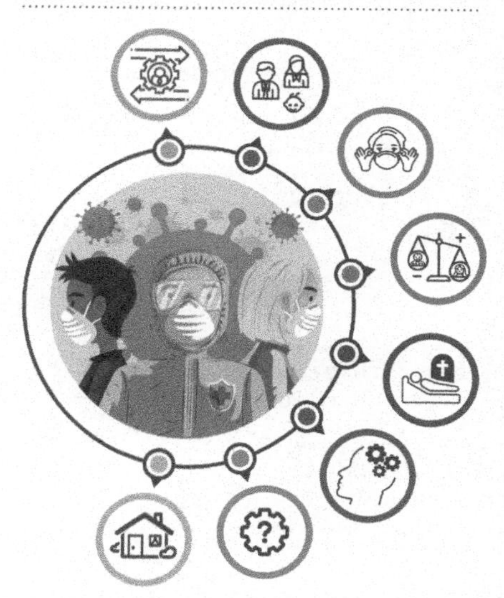

GUIDANCE
One source of concern included lack of guidance or rapidly changing guidance, particularly in relation to PPE.

WORKERS AND FAMILY
Healthcare workers (HCWs) were afraid of being exposed to the virus due to lack of adequate PPE and potentially infecting family members.

PPE
PPE was tiring, hot and uncomfortable and complicated communication with colleagues and patients.

INEQUALITIES
The burden of working on the frontlines disproportionately impacted women because women are overrepresented in lower-ranking jobs that are more likely to be redeployed to the frontlines, sometimes without sufficient training & adequate protection.

NEW ROLES IN RELATION TO DEATH
HCWs were forced to take on new roles accompanying patients at end of life due to family visiting restrictions and their desire to ensure patients did not die alone.

MENTAL HEALTH SUPPORT
HCWs reported an increased availability of formal mental health support, however, understaffing or clashing schedules prevented them from participating in these activities.

REDEPLOYMENT
Lack of training for redeployed staff and the failure to consider the skills of redeployed staff for new areas were identified as problems.

RECOVERING PATIENTS
COVID-19 is producing long term impairments and disabilities in recovering patients, and HCWs are concerned patient recovery may be prolonged due to unequal access to rehabilitation services.

POSITIVE ASPECTS OF DAILY WORK REPORTED BY HCWS INCLUDED SOLIDARITY BETWEEN COLLEAGUES, FEELING VALUED BY SOCIETY AND THE ABILITY TO PRODUCE RAPID CHANGES IN SERVICE DELIVERY (SUPPORTED BY HOSPITAL MANAGEMENT).

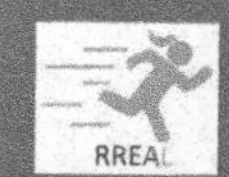

The studies are coordinated by the Rapid Research Evaluation and Appraisal Lab (RREAL):
Elysse Bautista Gonzalez, Caroline Buck, Georgia Chisnall, Silvie Cooper, Nehla Djellouli, Ginger Johnson, Louisa Manby, Franco Marquez, Lucy Mitchinson, Sofia Mulcahy Symmons, Georgina Singleton, Kirsi Sumray, Sasha Lewis-Jackson, Norha Vera, Anna Downick, Nina Regenold, Katarina Hoernke, Anna Badley, Hannah Robinson, Felicia Rand, Lily Andrews, Sam Martin, Sam Vanderslott, Harrison Fillmore, Laura Maio Aron Syversen and Cecilia Vindrola-Padros.
For more information, please contact Dr Cecilia Vindrola: c.vindrola@ucl.ac.uk

Figure 8.2 Infographic developed to share emerging findings with HCWs who took part in COVID-19 rapid qualitative study

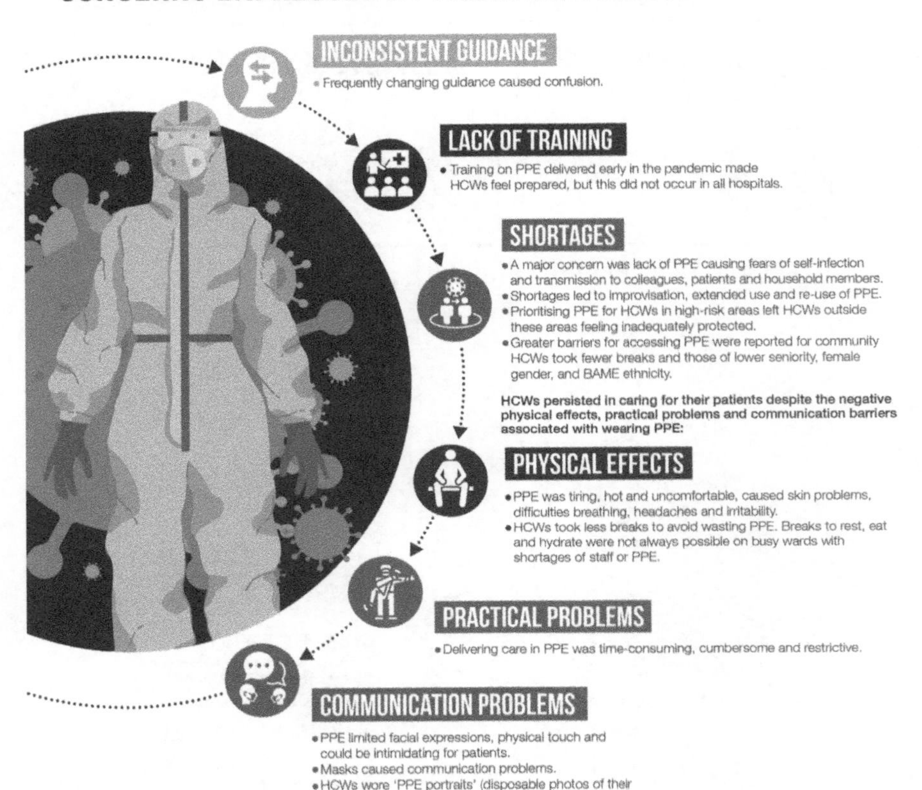

RREAL
Rapid Research Evaluation and Appraisal Lab
The study was carried out by Katarina Hoernke, Louisa Manby, Sam Martin, Samantha Vanderslott, Sasha Lewis-Jackson, Nehla Djellouli, and Cecilia Vindrola-Padros as part of the Rapid Research Evaluation and Appraisal Lab (RREAL).
Visual abstract design: Franco Marquez.
To read the full article, please visit: https://www.rapidresearchandevaluation.com/handouts

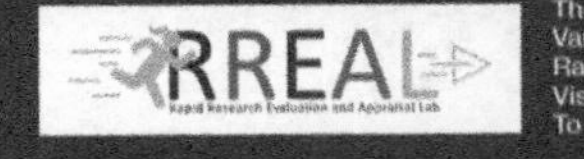

Figure 8.3 Visual abstract of our analysis on HCWs' experiences with PPE

to the studies that had been put on hold during the pandemic. We lost three researchers at the beginning of this month, who remained in touch via email in relation to the papers in development but did not participate in team meetings or take on additional pieces of work. We could no longer count on the graduate students who had submitted their theses and were now transitioning to other graduate programmes or jobs. All of them continued leading the papers that emerged from their theses but (with the exception of one student) did not engage in the other workstreams that were still ongoing. By the end of this month, we only had five researchers who continued as active members of this study (all senior researchers and all considered members of the RREAL core team).

Next Steps

We have started to develop an analytical plan for the two areas of focus we initially identified as being more long term: (1) an analysis of the different types of impact of the pandemic on HCWs' mental health and their change through time and (2) the analysis of HCWs' experiences in relation to inequalities produced by class and ethnicity. Our attention also shifted to survivorship and patients' access to care for rehabilitation services as well as HCWs' perceptions of vaccination.

At the moment, we are also having conversations with the organisations we have partnered with throughout the study to see how our final analysis of the findings and the long-term pieces of work identified above can be used to inform future planning in the NHS. These findings will be used to inform care delivery in the case of a second surge of cases as well as planning for future pandemics.

Discussion Questions

1. What were the main challenges the team faced when designing and implementing this study?
2. What were the main strategies developed by the team to address these challenges?
3. What other strategies (not mentioned in the chapter) do you think could have been used to address the same challenges?

Exercise 8

Rapid Appraisal

Considering the information provided in the rationale for the rapid appraisal section of this chapter, develop an alternative rapid appraisal design.

9

CASE STUDY 2: A RAPID SERVICE EVALUATION OF A PROGRAMME TO SUPPORT PARENTS OF CHILDREN WITH LEARNING DISABILITIES

In this chapter, I provide a detailed explanation of a rapid evaluation designed for a non-governmental organisation (NGO) that supported parents of children with learning disabilities. I include a detailed description of the study protocol (including a rapid literature review, a scoping phase and a qualitative process evaluation). I also discuss common challenges faced in rapid evaluations and the strategies our team used to address these.

Rationale for the Evaluation

The team was approached by the NGO because they were interested in documenting the implementation of a new approach, which relied on the active participation of members of the community (in this case, parents of children with learning disabilities). After considering the needs of the NGO and how they were planning to use the findings, the team proposed to carry out a formative process evaluation of the implementation of this participatory approach. The NGO was not clear on the scope of the evaluation and how they could use the evaluation findings to make changes in real time. Therefore, the team proposed to carry out a rapid literature review of similar approaches as well as a scoping study during the early stages of the project to clarify the scope and agree the research questions that would guide the evaluation. The study duration from scoping to the submission of a final report was nine months, with three feedback loops established throughout the duration of the study.

Workstreams

Scoping Study

The main outcome from the scoping study was the selection of areas to be included in the evaluation and agreement on the research questions, evaluation methods and dissemination plan. The research team used the findings from this scoping study to design the other streams of the evaluation.

Aims of the Scoping Study

1. Define the aims and areas covered in the evaluation.
2. Refine the research questions guiding the evaluation.
3. Outline the details of the study design (including the sampling framework).
4. Agree an evaluation timeline.
5. Agree the evaluation outputs, feedback processes and develop a dissemination plan.

Research Questions for the Scoping Study

1. What is the programme theory underpinning the programme? What are the proposed benefits of change? What are the expected outcomes?
2. Who are the main stakeholders of the programme?
3. What are the main components of the programme? Which components need to be included in the evaluation?
4. What are the main costs incurred in the delivery of the programme? Are there any areas where there might be cost savings?
5. How is the NGO currently measuring the impact of the programme?

Scoping Study Process

The scoping study included informal conversations with six key stakeholders to obtain information on the context, current state of the programme and key activities, observations during NGO team meetings (10 hours of observation) and a review of relevant documents. This information was used to guide a workshop with key stakeholders to prioritise areas for the evaluation and refine the research questions.

The workshop began with a description of what the research team considered to be a draft programme theory guiding the implementation of the programme. The team then presented the main activities involved in this draft programme theory and the areas that could potentially be covered during the scope of the evaluation. During the informal conversations with stakeholders, the research team had asked them about the questions they would like the evaluation to answer. These were presented to stakeholders and grouped according to general themes. All stakeholders at the meeting then engaged in a discussion about their views in relation to the selected areas and questions and the final scope was agreed.

The research team then proceeded to present a draft proposal of the design of the evaluation, asking stakeholders at the workshop questions about the relevance of the research questions, feasibility of the design and suitability of the dissemination plan. The process for managing the evaluation, including the frequency of meetings and the creation and membership of an Evaluation Steering Committee, was also discussed and agreed. The main task for the research team after this workshop was to develop a full proposal for the evaluation based on these discussions and share it with the stakeholders who attended the workshop to obtain their feedback and final approval before the evaluation could formally begin.

Scoping Study Timeline

- Month 1: Agreement of scoping study aims and process by all stakeholders
- Month 2: Data collection and analysis for the scoping study
- Month 2: Workshop with all stakeholders

Rapid Review of the Literature

The team conducted a rapid literature review of the use of similar participatory approaches in the context of learning disabilities following the approach for rapid evidence synthesis developed by Tricco et al. (2017). This rapid review method follows a systematic review approach but proposes adaptations to some of the steps to reduce the amount of time required to carry out the review (i.e. the use of large teams to review abstracts, full texts and extract data; in lieu of dual screening and selection, a percentage of excluded articles is reviewed by a second reviewer; and software can be used for data extraction and synthesis) (Tricco et al., 2017).

Due to the broad scope of the topic, the review was divided into two parts: (1) an evidence mapping exercise (Miake-Lye et al., 2016) to rapidly map the landscape on this topic and develop a formal search strategy to be used in the systematic review and (2) a systematic review of the literature on the use of participatory approaches in the context of learning disabilities, including grey literature and peer-reviewed articles.

The team used the Preferred Reporting Items for Systematic Reviews and Meta-Analysis (PRISMA) statement (Moher et al., 2009) to guide the reporting of the methods and findings.

Review Research Questions

The review was guided by the following questions:

1. How are these participatory approaches defined in the context of learning disabilities and what are their main components?
2. What are the main factors acting as barriers and enablers in the implementation of these approaches?
3. What are the lessons learnt when using these approaches in the context of learning disabilities?
4. Have these approaches been evaluated? If so, how and what are the main outcomes?
5. Does the implementation of these approaches vary by sector (i.e. health vs social care)?

Search Strategy

We used a phased search approach.

Phase 1 (evidence mapping)

The first phase was broad and included a series of search waves where search terms were gradually added based on the keywords used in the selected literature. These searches were carried out on Web of Science and TRIP to capture peer-reviewed articles and grey literature.

Phase 2

The second phase was targeted and used the search strategy developed in phase 1. The search included published literature found on multiple databases: MEDLINE, CINAHL PLUS, PsychInfo, ProQuest Social Science, TRIP and Web of Science. Results were combined into Mendeley and duplicates were removed. The reference lists of included articles were screened to identify additional relevant publications.

Selection

Following rapid review methodology, one researcher screened the articles in the title phase, and a second reviewer cross-checked exclusions in the abstract and full-text phases. Disagreements were discussed until consensus was reached. The inclusion criteria used for study selection were: (1) focus on the implementation of the participatory approach, (2) focus on the context of learning disabilities, (3) report on the findings of empirical studies or including information on implementation and/or evaluation and (4) published in English.

Data Extraction and Management

The included articles were analysed using a data extraction form developed in Research Electronic Data Capture (REDCap). The form was developed after the initial screening of full-text articles. It was then piloted independently by two researchers using a random sample of five articles. Disagreements were discussed until consensus was reached. The data extraction form was finalised based on the findings from the pilot.

Data Synthesis

Data were exported from REDCap and the main article characteristics were synthesised. The information entered in free text boxes was exported from REDCap and analysed using framework analysis (Gale et al., 2013). The initial categories for the framework were informed by our research questions but we were also sensitive to topics emerging from the data.

Quality Assessment

The Mixed Methods Appraisal Tool (MMAT) was used to assess the quality of the articles published in peer-reviewed journals and the AACODS checklist (authority, accuracy, coverage, objectivity, date, significance) was used for grey literature (Pace et al., 2012). Two researchers rated these articles independently. In cases of disagreement, the raters discussed their responses until consensus was reached. Inter-rater reliability was calculated using the kappa statistic (Landis and Koch, 1977).

Qualitative Process Evaluation

The team proposed to carry out a qualitative process evaluation of the implementation of the programme. The aim of this component of the evaluation was to understand how the programme was being implemented and identify lessons learned throughout implementation. This involved studying (1) the processes guiding the development and implementation of the different components of the programme and (2) gathering stakeholders' perceptions on these processes.

Research Questions

The evaluation was guided by the following research questions:

1. What is the programme theory underpinning the programme?
2. What are the barriers and facilitators encountered in implementation?
3. What are staff and users' experiences with the programme?
4. What is the impact of wider contextual factors in shaping implementation?

5 What perceived benefits, if any, does the programme have?
6 What are the lessons for implementing similar programmes across different contexts?

Study Design

The evaluation was designed as a rapid formative evaluation, where the research team collaborated closely with staff from the NGO and other stakeholders to develop and implement research on identified needs, and share formative feedback at regular intervals. Formative feedback included: (1) sharing the evolving understanding of the programme theory and suggested refinements; (2) providing 'real-time' insights on implementation; and (3) analysing staff views on the processes of implementation. While the team worked in close partnership with professionals and managers, the team implemented a series of strategies to retain critical distance in order for the evaluation to provide independent findings.

Data Collection and Sampling

Data collection was carried out via semi-structured interviews, non-participant observation and documentary analysis. Thirty semi-structured interviews were conducted at multiple organisational levels with NGO staff, users and other stakeholders. The interviews were audio-recorded, but the researchers also took notes and recorded the key findings on RAP sheets developed for the different groups included in the sample.

The sampling for the interviews was developed using purposive and snowballing approaches. A sampling framework, including the size of the sample and groups that were targeted for the interviews, can be found in Table 9.1.

Table 9.1. Sampling framework for telephone interviews

Participant	Target number of interviews
Senior non-governmental organisation (NGO) staff	3
NGO staff using the participatory approach	5
NGO staff not using the participatory approach	4
Users of NGO services (parents)	10
Partner NGOs	2
Community services	6
Total	***30***

The team also observed relevant planning and implementation meetings and activities, completing 60 hours of observation. By observing and analysing these meetings and activities, the team identified how processes of implementation were carried out in practice, how decisions in relation to implementation were negotiated and the factors that shaped organisational culture. The observations were recorded in the form of unstructured fieldnotes, and key findings were added to the RAP sheet on a regular basis. Documents were analysed to further develop an understanding of the project, the programme theory and how it changed, and track implementation of the project over time.

Data Analysis

Key findings from the observations, interviews and documentary analysis were added to the RAP sheet as the evaluation was ongoing and these were shared with stakeholders on a regular basis. Further analysis was carried out by importing the data from interviews, observations and documentary analysis into NVivo and analysed using framework analysis (Gale et al., 2013). The categories from the framework were informed by our research questions and new topics emerging throughout the study.

Recruitment

Our team approached potential participants via email, sending them a copy of the information sheet, which included details about the purpose, design, expectations, risks and benefits of the study. Potential participants were given 48 hours to decide if they would like to take part in the study. Those who decided to take part in the study were asked to sign and email the researcher a consent form. The researcher proceeded to arrange a telephone interview at a time that was convenient for the participants.

Outputs from the Evaluation

The evaluation allowed us to develop the following outputs:

1. Regular sharing of emerging findings (see timeline below)
2. Standard evaluation framework that the NGO could use internally for evaluating future services (after our evaluation ended)
3. A final report capturing wider lessons for the implementation of similar projects in other contexts
4. The dissemination of the evaluation findings in an accessible format, including two infographics and one animation

Evaluation Timeline

Months 1–2: Scoping study and first feedback session
Month 2: Beginning of rapid literature review
Month 3: Evaluation design and set-up
Month 4: Sharing of emerging findings from literature review
Months 4–7: Qualitative study data collection

Month 5: Feedback session with the NGO
Month 6: Feedback session with the NGO
Month 7: Qualitative study data analysis wrap-up
Month 8: Write up of final report and development of other outputs
Month 9: Submission of evaluation outputs to the NGO

Discussion Questions

1. Why do you think the team decided to carry out a scoping study for this evaluation?
2. What other methods of data collection would have been suitable for this evaluation?
3. How would the evaluation design have differed if, instead of a formative design, the team would have opted for one-time feedback at the end of the evaluation?

Exercise 9

Rapid evaluations

Considering the information provided in the rationale for the evaluation section of this chapter, develop an alternative rapid evaluation design.

10

THE FUTURE OF RAPID QUALITATIVE RESEARCH

I have frequently seen rapid qualitative study designs portrayed as recent innovations in the field of qualitative research. This depiction lacks accuracy and erases decades of work, learning and methodological experimentation. In this book, I have tried to pay tribute to the researchers who spent countless hours developing unique approaches for rapid research, sharing research findings in a timely way, so these could be used to inform changes in policy and practice. If we disregard the rich history of rapid qualitative research, we risk making the same mistakes over and over and not learning from lessons already available in the literature. We also run the risk of applying these approaches in unintended ways, diminishing their engagement with theory, increasing their level of instrumentality and severing their ties with traditions in the social sciences. The future development of the field of rapid qualitative research will depend on our efforts to improve these approaches without losing sight of their history.

A Future Agenda for the Field of Rapid Qualitative Research

There are a few key areas that I think will need to be considered in the near future to further develop the field of rapid qualitative research. These involve different aspects of research, from engagement with theory to more pragmatic aspects such as funding.

Rapid Qualitative Research as a Dynamic Field

As mentioned earlier in this book, the field of rapid qualitative research includes several approaches with overlapping features and several examples of cross-fertilisation. When designing studies, techniques used in these approaches can be combined. As new tools and techniques are created, it will be important to continue mapping where innovations are made and learn from these experiences. Without disregarding the importance of the historical roots mentioned above, it will be important to consider research as a changing practice.

Rapid Qualitative Research and Theory

Rapid research has often been described as instrumental, lacking critical perspectives and engagement with theory (Cupit et al., 2018). Authors have argued that a direct consequence of this perceived instrumentality has been the failure to shed light on the politics of knowledge production involved in research and the domination of positivist frameworks (Vougioukalou et al., 2019). Furthermore, there is a belief that rapid qualitative studies have mainly focused on delivering actionable findings to programme or service managers, and have failed to engage in critical discussions related to the assumptions guiding the programme/service, the research findings or both (Cupit et al., 2018).

When reviewing the literature on rapid qualitative research, I have also identified gaps in reporting, and one of these gaps is related to the theoretical frameworks guiding the study (Johnson and Vindrola-Padros, 2017; Vindrola-Padros and Vindrola-Padros, 2018). Whether this is a gap in reporting or a gap in design (in the sense that the researchers did not identify an explicit theoretical approach to inform their work) remains unknown. An important future step will be to encourage researchers to actively think about the ways in which theoretical approaches from different disciplines have shaped all stages of research and include clear descriptions of these in publications. An area that warrants future research is exploring whether engagement with theory is limited in more compressed study timeframes.

Rapid Qualitative Research and Reflexivity

Another assumption has been that rapid qualitative research will not be able to engage with reflexivity, that is, the 'researcher's critical account of their "self-location" (gender, class, ethnicity etc.), interests, pre-assumptions and life experiences and how these shape their relationships with study participants and the research process itself' (Vindrola-Padros and Vindrola-Padros, 2018). Many publications reporting findings from rapid qualitative studies have not integrated this critical reflection into the text, but, similarly to issues related to theoretical engagement, there is no reason why time pressures should preclude researchers from considering reflexivity as an integral part of the research process. In Chapter 6, I explore the different reflexive approaches developed for rapid qualitative research, including a technique for team-based reflexive practices.

In addition to this work, several authors have also found ways to be reflexive and still carry out timely research. For instance, Bikker et al. (2017) developed frequent team debriefing sessions where they could reflect on the research process and problems encountered during data collection. These discussions led to wider reflections about team dynamics and the study design. Armstrong and Armstrong (2018) developed a team reflexivity approach also based on team meetings occurring at different levels (data collection teams, regional teams and international teams). Researchers kept diaries to reflect on their experiences of fieldwork and they were discussed frequently across these different teams (Armstrong and Armstrong, 2018). The studies were mainly designed as rapid ethnographies. Questions still remain about the integration of reflexivity in other types of rapid qualitative research approaches.

The Formalisation of Training

The development of the field of rapid qualitative research will benefit from the integration of training on these approaches into formal programmes of study. Existing courses on research methods could include examples of rapid qualitative research approaches or courses on rapid research could be integrated into undergraduate and graduate social science and health, education, social work and other types of research programmes. Formal training on rapid qualitative research could help ensure that researchers are aware of the rich history of the field, the best ways to apply these approaches, cases when rapid study designs are not appropriate and the best ways to report the study design and findings.

The Sustainability of Research Teams

As mentioned earlier in the book, rapid qualitative research teams are often faced with issues regarding their sustainability if funding is obtained on a project by project basis. Teams will need to explore new ways of working and potentially rely on 'hybrid' models of funding. They might also need to rely on collaborations with other teams doing similar work to pool resources together in the case of larger projects. As rapid qualitative research becomes more mainstream, teams might become more successful with grant applications. However, funding bodies will need to revise their existing review and funding timelines to make sure these are suitable for rapid studies.

Rapid Qualitative Research Principles

Discussions on the assumptions between time and rigour, relationship-building, theory and reflexivity have raised important issues in relation to the production of knowledge in rapid qualitative research. Based on the main points described above and regardless of the diversity of rapid qualitative research approaches, I think an important starting point for the future development of the field will be reaching an agreement on the main principles that rapid qualitative studies share. An initial list could include:

- The researcher's perception of the social world under study is shaped by their own history, experiences, theoretical inclinations and the context under study, and will always be partial.
- The researcher also has an impact on the context and participants involved in the study as their presence is never neutral.
- Interpretations or meaning-making processes are carried out and negotiated with a wide range of stakeholders with multiple (and perhaps conflicting) views and interests.

- The development of relationships with study participants will lead to better insight and representation of their world views and realities.
- There is some level of pragmatism in rapid qualitative studies, in the sense that research is seen as leading to the crafting of data so these can be transformed into 'actionable findings'. The ultimate use of these findings to make changes in practice and policy will be shaped by a process of negotiation between the researcher and a wider range of stakeholders and will depend on the political interests of those involved. In other words, the knowledge generated in rapid qualitative studies cannot be considered independently of the context and relationships (including unequal power relations) that have shaped its production.
- The epistemological assumptions listed here might constitute core components of rapid qualitative research but, instead of being thought about in their purist form, it is important to consider them as continuously changing practices.

Rapid qualitative research approaches are becoming more popular and there has been an international drive to promote their use. The future of this field will depend on our ability to build global networks of researchers, research users, policymakers and practitioners, among others, interested in research that is timely, relevant and responsive. I hope this book can mark the start of these collaborations and pave the way for the exciting future of rapid qualitative research that lies ahead.

Chapter Summary

- The future development of the field of rapid qualitative research will need to take into consideration the rich history of these approaches while seeking to generate innovation.
- There is a dominant assumption in qualitative research between time (or the duration of the study) and the rigour of a study.
- A detailed analysis of the field of rapid qualitative research points to the fact that rapid studies are also able to generate in-depth data, include the development of meaningful relationships with research participants, and engage with theory and reflexivity.
- The infrastructure of the field of rapid qualitative research will need to be strengthened by paying closer attention to the formalisation of training and sustainability of rapid research teams.

Discussion Questions

1. What are the underlying assumptions behind the association of time, theory and reflexivity in rapid qualitative research?
2. What are the challenges that still remain in the development of the field of rapid qualitative research?
3. Can you think of any future areas of development that have not been mentioned in this chapter?

Exercise 10

Theoretical Frameworks and the Researcher's Gaze

Option A

Think about your study topic and identify two different theoretical frameworks that could be used to guide the study and answer the following questions:

1. How would each framework shape the research questions?
2. What are the key factors you would need to pay attention to during data collection and how would these vary by framework?
3. How would these theoretical frameworks shape the analytical framework?

Option B

Read the description of the rapid qualitative study presented in Chapter 8. Identify two different theoretical frameworks that could have been used to guide the study and answer the following questions:

1. How would each framework shape the research questions?
2. What are the main aspects of HCWs' experiences of delivering care during the COVID-19 pandemic that the research team would have focused on during data collection? How would this have varied depending on the theoretical framework?
3. How would these theoretical frameworks shape the analytical framework?

APPENDIX 1: ADDITIONAL RESOURCES

Rapid Evaluation and Appraisal Methods (REAM) (Presenting General Overviews)

Anker, M., Guidotti, S., Orseszyna, S., & Thuroax, M. (1993). Rapid evaluation methods (REM) of health service performance: Methodological observations. *Bulletin of the World Health Organization, 71*(1), 15–21.

McNall, M. A., & Foster-Fishman, P. (2007). Methods of rapid evaluation, assessment, and appraisal. *American Journal of Evaluation, 28*(2), 151–168. https://doi.org/10.1177/1098214007300895

McNall, M. A., Welch, V. E., Ruh, K. L., Mildner, C. A., & Soto, T. (2004). The use of rapid-feedback evaluation methods to improve the retention rates of an HIV/AIDS healthcare intervention. *Evaluation and Program Planning, 27*, 287–294. https://doi.org/10.1016/j.evalprogplan.2004.04.003

Nunns, H. (2009). Responding to the demand for quicker evaluation findings. *Social Policy Journal of New Zealand, 34*, 89–99.

Shrank, W. (2013). The center for medicare and medicaid innovation's blueprint for rapid-cycle evaluation of new care and payment models. *Health Affairs, 32*, 807–812. https://doi.org/10.1377/hlthaff.2013.0216

Systematic Literature Reviews

Johnson, G., & Vindrola-Padros, C. (2017). Rapid qualitative research methods during complex health emergencies: A systematic review of the literature. *Social Science and Medicine, 189*, 63–75. https://doi.org/10.1016/j.socscimed.2017.07.029

Vindrola-Padros, C., Brage, E., & Johnson, G. A. (2021). Rapid, responsive and relevant? A systematic review of rapid evaluations in healthcare. *American Journal of Evaluation, 42*(1), 13–27. https://doi.org/10.1177/1098214019886914

Vindrola-Padros, C., & Jonhson, G. A. (2020). Rapid techniques in qualitative research: A critical review of the literature. *Qualitative Health Research, 30*(10), 1596–1604. https://doi.org/10.1177/1049732320921835

Vindrola-Padros, C., & Vindrola-Padros, B. (2018). Quick and dirty? A systematic review of the use of rapid ethnographies in healthcare organisation and delivery. *BMJ Quality and Safety, 27*, 321–330. https://doi.org/10.1136/bmjqs-2017-007226

Rapid Appraisals, Rapid Qualitative Inquiry (RQI), Rapid Assessment Procedures and Process (RAP) and the RARE Model

Abramowitz, S., McLean, K. E., McKune, S. L., Bardosh, K. L., Fallah, M., Monger, J., & Tehoungue, K. (2015). Community-centered responses to Ebola in urban Liberia: The view from below. *PLOS Neglected Tropical Diseases, 9*(4), e0003706. https://doi.org/10.1371/journal.pntd.0003706

Beebe, J. (1995). Basic concepts and techniques of rapid appraisal. *Human Organization, 54*(1), 42–51. https://doi.org/10.17730/humo.54.1.k84tv883mr2756l3

Beebe, J. (2001). *Rapid assessment process: An introduction*. Altamira Press.

Beebe, J. (2005). Rapid assessment process. In K. Kempf-Leonard (Ed.), *Encyclopedia of social measurement* (pp. 285–291). Elsevier.

Beebe, J. (2014). *Rapid qualitative inquiry* (2nd ed.). Rowman and Littlefield.

Brown, D., Hernández, A., Saint-Jean, G., Evans, S., Tafari, I., Brewster, L. G., & Akal, S. (2008). A participatory action research pilot study of urban health disparities using rapid assessment response and evaluation. *American Journal of Public Health, 98*(1), 28–38. https://doi.org/10.2105/AJPH.2006.091363

Chambers, R. (1994a). Participatory rural appraisal: Analysis of experience. *World Development, 22*(9), 1253–1268. https://doi.org/10.1016/0305-750X(94)90003-5

Chambers, R. (1994b). The origins and practice of participatory rural appraisal. *World Development, 22*(7), 953–969. https://doi.org/10.1016/0305-750X(94)90141-4

Fitch, C., Rhodes, T., & Stimson, G. (2000). Origins of an epidemic: The methodological and political emergence of rapid assessment. *International Journal of Drug Policy, 11*, 63–82. https://doi.org/10.1016/S0955-3959(99)00056-0

Harris, K., Jerome, N., & Fawcett, S. (1997). Rapid assessment procedures: A review and critique. *Human Organization, 56*(3), 375–378. https://doi.org/10.17730/humo.56.3.w525025611458003

Manderson, L., & Aaby, P. (1992a). Can rapid anthropological procedures be applied to tropical diseases? *Health Policy and Planning, 7*(1), 46–55. https://doi.org/10.1093/heapol/7.1.46

Manderson, L., & Aaby, P. (1992b). An epidemic in the field? Rapid assessment procedures and health research. *Social Science and Medicine, 35*(7), 839–850. https://doi.org/10.1016/0277-9536(92)90098-B

McMullen, C., Ash, J. S., Sittig, D. F., Bunce, A., Guappone, K., Dykstra, R., & Wright, A. (2011). Rapid assessment of clinical information systems in the healthcare setting: An efficient method for time-pressed evaluation. *Methods of Information in. Medicine, 50*(4), 299–307. https://doi.org/10.3414/ME10-01-0042

Rifkin, S. (1992). Rapid appraisals for health: An overview. *Rapid Rural Appraisal Notes, 16*, 7–12.

Scrimshaw, S., & Hurtado, E. (1988). Anthropological involvement on the Central American diarrheal disease control project. *Social Science and Medicine, 27*(1), 97–105. https://doi.org/10.1016/0277-9536(88)90167-0

Trotter, R. T. II., Needle, R. H., Goosby, E., Bates, C., & Singer, M. (2001). A methodological model for rapid assessment, response, and evaluation: The RARE program in public health. *Field Methods, 13*(2), 137–159. https://doi.org/10.1177/1525822X0101300202

Utarini, A., Winkvist, A., & Pelto, G. (2001). Appraising studies in health using rapid assessment procedures (RAP): Eleven critical criteria. *Human Organization, 60*(4), 390–400. https://doi.org/10.17730/humo.60.4.3xu3p85amf13avtp

Rapid Ethnographies (General Descriptions of the Approach)

Bentley, M., Pelto, G., Straus, W., Schumann, D., Adegbola, C., Pena, de la, & Huffman, S. L. (1988). Rapid ethnographic assessment: Applications in diarrhea management program. *Social Science and Medicine, 27*(1), 107–116. https://doi.org/10.1016/0277-9536(88)90168-2

Cruz, E., & Higginbottom, G. (2013). The use of focused ethnography in nursing research. *Nurse Researcher, 20*(4), 36–43. https://doi.org/10.7748/nr2013.03.20.4.36.e305

Handwerker, P. (2001). *Quick ethnography: A guide to rapid multi-method research*. AltaMira Press.

Knoblauch, H. (2005). Focused ethnography. *Forum: Qualitative Social Research, 6*(3), 1–14.

Pink, S., & Morgan, J. (2013). Short-term ethnography: Intense routes to knowing. *Symbolic Interaction, 36*(3), 351–361. https://doi.org/10.1002/symb.66

Rapid Tools to Speed Up Data Collection or Analysis

Anderson, J. (1998). Transcribing with voice recognition software: A new tool for qualitative researchers. *Qualitative Health Research, 8*(5), 718–723. https://doi.org/10.1177/104973239800800511

Burgess-Allen, J., & Owen-Smith, V. (2010). Using mind mapping techniques for rapid qualitative data analysis in public participation processes. *Health Expect, 13*, 406–415. https://doi.org/10.1111/j.1369-7625.2010.00594.x

Gravois, T., Rosenfield, S., & Greenberg, B. (1992). Establishing reliability for coding implementation concerns of school-based teams from audiotapes. *Evaluation Review, 16*(5), 562–569. https://doi.org/10.1177/0193841X9201600507

Greenwood, M., Kendrick, T., Davies, H., & Gill, F. (2017). Hearing voices: Comparing two methods for analysis of focus group data. *Applied Nursing Research, 35*, 90–93. https://doi.org/10.1016/j.apnr.2017.02.024

Halcomb, E. J., & Davidson, P. M. ((2006). February). Is verbatim transcription of interview data always necessary? *Applied Nursing Research, 19*(1), 38–42. https://doi.org/10.1016/j.apnr.2005.06.001

Joe, J., Chaudhuri, S., Le, T., Thompson, H., & Demiris, G. (2015). The use of think-aloud and instant data analysis in evaluation research: Exemplar and lessons learned. *Journal of Biomedical Informatics, 56*, 284–291. https://doi.org/10.1016/j.jbi.2015.06.001

Johnson, B. (2011). The speed and accuracy of voice recognition software-assisted transcription versus the listen-and-type method: A research note. *Qualitative Research, 11*(1), 91–97. https://doi.org/10.1177/1468794110385966

Lopez, K. D., Febretti, A., Stifter, J., Johnson, A., Wilkie, D. J., & Keenan, G. (2017, October). Toward a more robust and efficient usability testing method of clinical decision support for nurses derived from nursing electronic health record data. *International Journal of Nursing Knowledge, 28*(4), 211–218. https://doi.org/10.1111/2047-3095.12146

Markle, T., West, R., & Rich, P. (2011). Beyond transcription: Technology, change and refinement of method. *Forum: Qualitative Social Research, 12*(3), art. 21.

Neal, J., Neal, Z., VanDyke, E., & Kornbluh, M. (2015). Expediting the analysis of qualitative data in evaluation: A procedure for the rapid identification of themes from audio recordings (RITA). *American Journal of Evaluation, 36*(1), 118–132. https://doi.org/10.1177/1098214014536601

Park, J., & Zeanah, E. (2005). An evaluation of voice recognition software for use in interview-based research: A research note. *Qualitative Research, 5*(2), 245–251. https://doi.org/10.1177/1468794105050837

Petro, N. (2010). Hate taking notes? Try mind mapping. *GP Solo, 27*(4), 20–23. https://www.jstor.org/stable/23630192

Scott, S. D., Sharpe, H., O'Leary, K., Dehaeck, U., Hindmarsh, K., Moore, J. G., & Osmond, M. H. ((2009). January). Court reporters: A viable solution for the challenges of focus group data collection? *Qualitative Health Research, 19*(1), 140–146. https://doi.org/10.1177/1049732308327883

Tattersall, C., & Vernon, S. (2007). Mind mapping as a tool in qualitative research. *Nursing Times, 103*(26), 32–33.

Taylor, B., Henshall, C., Kenyon, S., Litchfield, I., & Greenfield, S. (2018). Can rapid approaches to qualitative analysis deliver timely, valid findings to clinical leaders? A mixed methods study comparing rapid and thematic analysis. *BMJ Open, 8*(10), e019993. https://doi.org/10.1136/bmjopen-2017-019993

Tessier, S. (2012). From field notes to transcripts to tape recordings: Evolution or combination? *International Journal of Qualitative Methods, 11*(4), 446–460. https://doi.org/10.1177/160940691201100410

Watkins, D. (2017). Rapid and rigorous qualitative data analysis: The 'RADaR' Technique for applied research. *International Journal of Qualitative Methods, 16*, 1–9. https://doi.org/10.1177/1609406917712131

Rapid Evaluations

Anker, M., Guidotti, R. J., Orzeszyna, S., Sapirie, S. A., & Thuriaux, M. C. (1993). Rapid evaluation methods (REM) of health services performance: Methodological observations. *Bulletin of the World Health Organization, 71*(1), 15–21.

Aspray, T. J., Nesbit, K., Cassidy, T. P., & Hawthorne, G. (2006). Rapid assessment methods used for health-equity audit: Diabetes mellitus among frail British care-home residents. *Public Health, 120*(11), 1042–1051. https://doi.org/10.1016/j.puhe.2006.06.002

Bjornson-Benson, W. M., Stibolt, T. B., Manske, K. A., Zavela, K. J., Youtsey, D. J., & Buist, A. S. (1993). Monitoring recruitment effectiveness and cost in a clinical trial. *Controlled Clinical Trials, 14*(Suppl. 2), 52S–67S. https://doi.org/10.1016/0197-2456(93)90024-8

Chowdhury, S. N. M., & Moni, D. (2004). A situation analysis of the menstrual regulation programme in Bangladesh. *Reproductive Health Matters, 12*(Suppl. 24), 95–104. https://doi.org/10.1016/S0968-8080(04)24020-4

Felisberto, E., Freese, E., Natal, S., & Alves, C. K. (2008). A contribution to institutionalized health evaluation: A proposal for self-evaluation. *Cadernos de saude publica, 24*(9), 2091–2102. https://doi.org/10.1590/S0102-311X2008000900015

Gale, R., Wu, J., Erhardt, T., Bounthavong, M., Reardon, C., Damschroder, L., & Midboe, A. (2019). Comparison of rapid vs in-depth qualitative analytic methods from a process evaluation of academic detailing in the Veterans Health Administration. *Implementation Science, 14,* 11. https://doi.org/10.1186/s13012-019-0853-y

Glasgow, R., Kessler, R. S., Ory, M. G., Roby, D., Gorin, S. S., & Krist, A. (2014). Conducting rapid, relevant research lessons learned from the My Own Health Report project. *American Journal of Preventive Medicine, 47*(2), 212–219. https://doi.org/10.1016/j.amepre.2014.03.007

Grant, L., Brown, J., Leng, M., Bettega, N., & Murray, S. A. (2011). Palliative care making a difference in rural Uganda, Kenya and Malawi: Three rapid evaluation field studies. *BMC Palliative Care, 10,* 8. https://doi.org/10.1186/1472-684X-10-8

Grasso, P. (2003). What makes an evaluation useful? Reflections from experience in large organizations. *American Journal of Evaluation, 24*(4), 507–514. https://doi.org/10.1177/109821400302400408

Keith, R. (2017). Using the consolidated framework for implementation research (CFIR) to produce actionable findings: A rapid-cycle evaluation approach to improving implementation. *Implementation Science, 12,* 15. https://doi.org/10.1186/s13012-017-0550-7

McNall, M., Welch, V., Ruh, K., Mildner, C., & Soto, T. (2004). The use of rapid-feedback evaluation methods to improve the retention rates of an HIV/AIDS healthcare intervention. *Evaluation and Program Planning, 27,* 287–294. https://doi.org/10.1016/j.evalprogplan.2004.04.003

Munday, D., Haraldsdottir, E., Manak, M., & Thyle, A. (2018). Rural palliative care in North India: Rapid evaluation of a program using a realist mixed method approach. *Indian Journal of Palliative Care, 24*(1), 3–8.

Nunns, H. (2009). Responding to the demand for quicker evaluation findings. *Social Policy Journal of New Zealand, 34,* 89–99.

Riley, W., Glasgow, R. E., Etheredge, L., & Abernethy, A. P. (2013). Rapid, responsive, relevant (R3) research: A call for a rapid learning health research enterprise. *Clinical and Translational Science, 2,* 10. https://doi.org/10.1186/2001-1326-2-10

Sandison, P. (2003). *Desk-based review of real-time evaluation experience.* UNICEF.

Schneeweiss, S., Shrank, W. H., Ruhl, M., & Maclure, M. (2015). Decision-making aligned with rapid-cycle evaluation in health care. *International Journal of Technology Assessment in Health Care, 31,* 214–222. https://doi.org/10.1017/S0266462315000410

Shrank, W. (2013). The Center for Medicare and Medicaid Innovation's blueprint for rapid-cycle evaluation of new care and payment models. *Health Affairs, 32*(4), 807–812. https://doi.org/10.1377/hlthaff.2013.0216

Skillman, M., Cross-Barnet, C., Singer, R. F., Rotondo, C., Ruiz, S., & Moiduddin, A. (2019). A framework for rigorous qualitative research as a component of mixed method rapid-cycle evaluation. *Qualitative Health Research, 29*(2), 279–289. https://doi.org/10.1177/1049732318795675

Taylor, B., Henshall, C., Kenyon, S., Litchfield, I., & Greenfield, S. (2018). Can rapid approaches to qualitative analysis deliver timely, valid findings to clinical leaders? A mixed methods study comparing rapid and thematic analysis. *BMJ Open, 8,* e019993. https://doi.org/10.1136/bmjopen-2017-019993

Zakocs, R., Hill, J. A., Brown, P., Wheaton, J., & Freire, K. E. (2015). The data-to-action framework: A rapid program improvement process. *Health Education & Behavior: The Official Publication of the Society for Public Health Education, 42*(4), 471–479. https://doi.org/10.1177/1090198115595010

Rapid Ethnographies

Ackerman. S. L., Sarkar, U., Tieu, L., Handley, M. A., Schillinger, D., Hahn, K., & Lyles, C. (2017, March 15). Meaningful use in the safety net: A rapid ethnography of patient portal implementation at five community health centers in California. *Journal of the American Medical Informatics Association, 24*(5), 903–912. https://doi.org/10.1093/jamia/ocx015

Armstrong, P., & Lowndes, R. (Eds). (2018). *Creative teamwork: Developing rapid, site-switching ethnography*. Oxford University Press.

Baines, D., & Cunningham, I. (2011). Using comparative perspective rapid ethnography in international case studies: Strengths and challenges. *Qualitative Social Work, 12*(1), 73–88. https://doi.org/10.1177/1473325011419053

Brown-Johnson, C., Shaw, J., Safaeinilli, N., Chan, G., Mahoney, M., Asch, S., & Winget, M. (2019). Role definition is key? Rapid qualitative ethnography findings from a team-based primary care transformation. *Learning Health Systems, 3*(3), e10188. https://doi.org/10.1002/lrh2.10188

Charlesworth, S., & Baines, D. (2015). Understanding the negotiation of paid and unpaid care work in community services in cross-national perspective: the contribution of a rapid ethnographic approach. *Journal of Family Studies, 21*(1), 7–21. https://doi.org/10.1080/13229400.2015.1010263

Chesluk, B. J., Bernabeo, E., Reddy, S., Lynn, L., Hess, B., Odhner, T., & Holmboe, E. (2015). How hospitalists work to pull healthcare teams together. *Journal of Health Organization and Management, 29*(7), 933–947. https://doi.org/10.1108/JHOM-01-2015-0008

Chesluk, B. J., & Holmboe, E. S. (2010, May). How teams work – or don't – in primary care: A field study on internal medicine practices. *Health Affairs, 29*(5), 874–879. https://doi.org/10.1377/hlthaff.2009.1093

Choy, I., Kitto, S., Adu-aryee, N., & Okrainec, A. (2013, November). Barriers to the uptake of laparoscopic surgery in a lower-middle-income country. *Surgical Endoscopy, 27*(11), 4009–4015. https://doi.org/10.1007/s00464-013-3019-z

Culhane-Pera, K. A., Sriphetcharawut, S., Thawsirichuchai, R., Yangyuenkun, W., & Kunstadter, P. (2015, November). Afraid of delivering at the hospital or afraid of delivering at home: A qualitative study of Thai Hmong families' decision-making about maternity services. *Maternal and Child Health Journal, 19*(11), 2384–2392. https://doi.org/10.1007/s10995-015-1757-3

Ferreira, S., Sayagob, S., & Blatc, J. (2016). Going beyond telecenters to foster the digital inclusion of older people in Brazil: Lessons learned from a rapid ethnographical study. *Information Technology for Development, 22*(S1), 26–46. https://doi.org/10.1080/02681102.2015.1091974

Halme, M., Kourula, A., Lindeman, S., Kallio, G., & Lima-Toivanen, M. (2016). Sustainability innovation at the base of the pyramid through multi-sited rapid ethnography. *Corporate Social Responsibility and Environmental Management, 23*, 113–128. https://doi.org/10.1002/csr.1385

Hussain, R. S., McGarvey, S. T., & Fruzzetti, L. M. (2015, March). Partition and poliomyelitis: An investigation of the Polio disparity affecting Muslims during India's eradication program. *PLOS ONE, 10*(3), n/a. https://doi.org/10.1371/journal.pone.0115628

Jayawardena, A., Wijayasinghe, S. R., Tennakoon, D., Cook, T., & Morcuende, J. A. (2013). Early effects of a 'train the trainer' approach to Ponseti method dissemination: A case study of Sri Lanka. *Iowa Orthopedic Journal, 33*, 153–160.

Kluwin, T., Morris, C., & Clifford, J. (2004). A rapid ethnography of itinerant teachers of the deaf. *American Annals of the Deaf, 149*(1), 62–72. https://doi.org/10.1353/aad.2004.0012

McElroy, T., Konde-Lule, J., Neema, S., & Gitta, S. (2007, June 15–30). Uganda sustainable clubfoot care. Understanding the barriers to clubfoot treatment adherence in Uganda: A rapid ethnographic study. *Disability and Rehabilitation, 29*(11–12), 845–855. https://doi.org/10.1080/09638280701240102

McKeown, M., Thomson, G., Scholes, A., Edgar, F., Downe, S., Price, O., & Duxbury, J. (2019). Restraint minimisation in mental health care: Legitimate or illegitimate force? An ethnographic study. *Sociology of Health and Illness, 42*(3), 449–464. https://doi.org/10.1111/1467-9566.13015

Mignone, J., Hiremath, G., Sabni, V., Laxmi, B., Halli, S., O'Neil, J., & Moses, S. (2009). Use of rapid ethnographic methodology to develop a village-level rapid assessment tool predictive of HIV infection in rural India. *International Journal of Qualitative Methods, 8*(3), 52–67.

Millen, D. (2000). *Rapid ethnography: Time deepening strategies for HCI*. Field Research.

Mudiyanselage, N. (2017). 'Rapid' but not 'raid': A reflection on the use of rapid ethnography in entrepreneurship research. *Qualitative Research Journal, 17*(4), 254–264. https://doi.org/10.1108/QRJ-12-2015-0098

Saleem, J. J., Plew, W. R., Speir, R. C., Herout, J., Wilck, N. R., Ryan, D. M., & Phillips, T. (2015, July). Understanding barriers and facilitators to the use of clinical information systems for intensive care units and anesthesia record keeping: A rapid ethnography. *International Journal of Medical Informatics, 84*(7), 500–511. https://doi.org/10.1016/j.ijmedinf.2015.03.006

Schwitters, A., Lederer, P., Zilversmit, L., Gudo, P. S., Ramiro, I., Cumba, L., & Jobarteh, K. (2015, March 5). Barriers to health care in rural Mozambique: a rapid ethnographic assessment of planned mobile health clinics for ART. *Global Health: Science and Practice, 3*(1), 109–116. https://doi.org/10.9745/GHSP-D-14-00145

Quick Ethnographies

Mullaney, T., Pettersson, H., Nyholm, T., & Stolterman, E. (2012, December). Thinking beyond the cure: A case for human-centered design in cancer care. *International Journal of Design, 6*(3), www.ijdesign.org/index.php/IJDesign/article/view/1076

Focused Ethnographies

Andreassen, P., Christensen, M., & Møller, J. (2019). Focused ethnography as an approach in medical education research. *Medical Education, 54*(4), 296–302. https://doi.org/10.1111/medu.14045

Bikker, A., Atherton, H., Brant, H., Porqueddu, T., Campbell, J., Gibson, A., & Ziebland, S. (2017). Conducting a team-based multi-sited focused ethnography in primary care. *BMC Medical Research Methodology, 17*, 139. https://doi.org/10.1186/s12874-017-0422-5

Conte, K. P., Shahid, A., Grøn, S., Loblay, V., Green, A., Innes-Hughes, C., & Persson, L. (2019). Capturing implementation knowledge: Applying focused ethnography to study how implementers generate and manage knowledge in the scale-up of obesity prevention programs. *Implementation Science, 14*, 91. https://doi.org/10.1186/s13012-019-0938-7

Dupuis-Blanchard, S., Neufeld, A., & Strang, V. T. (2009). The significance of social engagement in relocated older adults. *Qualitative Health Research, 19*(9), 1186–1195. https://doi.org/10.1177/1049732309343956

Ensign, J., & Bell, M. (2004). Illness experiences of homeless youth. *Qualitative Health Research, 14*(9), 1239–1254. https://doi.org/10.1177/1049732304268795

Gagnon, A. J., Carnevale, F., & Mehta, P. (2013). Developing population interventions with migrant women for maternal-child health: A focused ethnography. *BMC Public Health, 13*, 471. https://doi.org/10.1186/1471-2458-13-471

Garcia, C., & Saewyc, E. (2007). Perceptions of mental health among recently immigrated Mexican adolescents. *Issues in Mental Health Nursing, 28*(1), 37–54. https://doi.org/10.1080/01612840600996257

Higginbottom, G. M. A. (2011). The transitioning experiences of internationally-educated nurses into a Canadian health care system: A focused ethnography. *BMC Nursing, 10*(14), 1–13. https://doi.org/10.1186/1472-6955-10-14

Kilian, C., Salmoni, A., Ward-Griffin, C., & Kloseck, M. (2008). Perceiving falls within a family context: A focused ethnographic approach. *Canadian Journal on Aging, 27*(4), 331–345. https://doi.org/10.3138/cja.27.4.331

Kitchen, C. E. W., Lewis, S., Tiffin, P. A., Welsh, P. R., Howey, L., & Ekers, D. (2017). A focused ethnography of a child and adolescent mental health service: Factors relevant to the implementation of a depression trial. *Trials, 18*, 237. https://doi.org/10.1186/s13063-017-1982-8

Mason, B., Epiphaniou, E., Nanton, V., Donaldson, A., Shipman, C., Daveson, B. A., & Murray, S. A. (2013). Coordination of care for individuals with advanced progressive conditions: A multi-site ethnographic and serial interview study. *British Journal of General Practice, 63*(613), e580–e588. https://doi.org/10.3399/bjgp13X670714

Pasco, A. C., Morse, J. M., & Olson, J. K. (2004). The cross-cultural relationships between nurses and Filipino Canadian patients. *Journal of Nursing Scholarship, 36*(3), 239–246. https://doi.org/10.1111/j.1547-5069.2004.04044.x

Patmon, F., Gee, P., Rylee, T., & Readdy, N. (2016). Using interactive patient engagement technology in clinical practice: A qualitative assessment of nurses' perceptions. *Journal of Medical Internet Research, 18*(11), 30–42. https://doi.org/10.2196/jmir.5667

Plaza del Pino, F. J., Soriano, E., & Higginbottom, G. M. (2013). Sociocultural and linguistic boundaries influencing intercultural communication between nurses and Moroccan patients in southern Spain: A focused ethnography. *BMC Nursing, 12*, 14. https://doi.org/10.1186/1472-6955-12-14

Scott, S. D., & Pollock, C. (2008). The role of nursing unit culture in shaping research utilization behaviors. *Research in Nursing and Health, 31*(4), 298–309. https://doi.org/10.1002/nur.20264

Skårås, M. (2018). Focused ethnographic research on teaching and learning in conflict zones: History education in South Sudan. *Forum for Development Studies, 45*(2), 217–238. https://doi.org/10.1080/08039410.2016.1202316

Smallwood, A. (2009). Cardiac assessment teams: A focused ethnography of nurses' roles. *British Journal of Cardiac Nursing, 4*(3), 132–139. https://doi.org/10.12968/bjca.2009.4.3.40050

Spiers, J. A., & Wood, A. (2010). Building a therapeutic alliance in brief therapy: The experience of community mental health nurses. *Archives of Psychiatric Nursing, 24*(6), 373–386. https://doi.org/10.1016/j.apnu.2010.03.001

Tzeng, W. C., Yang, C. I., Tzeng, N. S., Ma, H. S., & Chen, L. (2010). The inner door: toward an understanding of suicidal patients. *Journal of Clinical Nursing, 19*(9–10), 1396–1404. https://doi.org/10.1111/j.1365-2702.2009.03002.x

Short-Term Ethnographies

Harte, J. D., Sheehan, A., Stewart, S. C., & Foureur, M. (2016, April). Childbirth supporters' experiences in a built hospital birth environment. *HERD: Health Environments Research & Design Journal, 9*(3), 135–161. https://doi.org/10.1177/1937586715622006

Rapid Systematic Reviews or Evidence Syntheses

Tricco, A., Antony, J., Zarin, W., Strifler, L., Ghassemi, M., & Ivory, J. (2015). A scoping review of rapid review methods. *BMC Medicine, 13*, 224. https://doi.org/10.1186/s12916-015-0465-6

Tricco, A., Langlois, E., & Straus, S. (2017). *Rapid reviews to strengthen health policy and systems: A practical guide*. Geneva: World Health Organization.

REFERENCES

Abramowitz, S. A., McLean, K. E., McKune, S. L., Bardosh, K. L., Fallah, M., Monger, J., & Omidian, P. A. (2015). Community-centered responses to Ebola in urban Liberia: The view from below. *PLOS Neglected Tropical Diseases, 9*(4), e0003706. http://dx.doi.org/10.1371/journal.pntd.0003706

Ackerman, S. L., Sarkar, U., Tieu, L., Handley, M. A., Schillinger, D., Hahn, K., & . . .Lyles, C. (2017). Meaningful use in the safety net: A rapid ethnography of patient portal implementation at five community health centers in California. *Journal of the American Medical Informatics Association, 24*(5), 903–912. http://dx.doi.org/10.1093/jamia/ocx015

Agyepong, I. A., Aryee, B., Dzikunu, H., & Manderson, L. (1995). *The Malaria Manual. Guidelines for the Rapid Assessment of Social, Economic and Cultural Aspects of Malaria.* Geneva: WHO.

Agyepong, I. A., & Manderson, L. (1994). The diagnosis and management of fever at household level in the Greater Accra Region, Ghana. *Acta Tropica, 58*(3–4), 317–330.

Anker, M., Guidotti, S., Orseszyna, S., & Thuroax, M. (1993). Rapid evaluation methods (REM) of health service performance: Methodological observations. *Bulletin of the World Health Organization, 71*(1), 15–21.

Aral, S., St. Lawrence, J., & Dyatlov, R. (2005). Commercial sex work, drug use, and sexually transmitted infections in St. Petersburg, Russia. *Social Science & Medicine, 60,* 2181–2190. https://doi.org/10.1016/j.socscimed.2004.10.009

Arksey, H., & O'Malley, L. (2005). Scoping studies: Towards a methodological framework. *International Journal of Social Research Methodology, 8,* 19–32. https://doi.org/10.1080/1364557032000119616

Armstrong, P., & Armstrong, H. (2018). Theory matters. In P. Armstrong & R. Lowndes (Eds), *Creative Teamwork: Developing Rapid, Site-Switching Ethnography* (pp. 1–20). Oxford University Press.

Armstrong, P., & Lowndes, R. (2018). *Creative Teamwork: Developing Rapid, Site-Switching Ethnography*. Oxford University Press.

Ash, J. S., Sittig, D. F., Dykstra, R. H., Wright, A., McMullen, C. K., Richardson, J. E., & Middleton, B. (2010). Identifying best practices for clinical decision support and knowledge management in the field. *Studies in Health Technology and Informatics, 160*(Pt 2), 806–810.

Ash, J. S., Sittig, D. F., Guappone, K. P., Dykstra, R. H., Richardson, J., Wright, A., & Middleton, B. (2012). Recommended practices for computerized clinical decision support and knowledge management in community settings: A qualitative study. *BMC Medical Informatics and Decision Making, 12*(1), 6. https://doi.org/10.1186/1472-6947-12-6

Aspray, T. J., Nesbit, K., Cassidy, T. P., & Hawthorne, G. (2006). Rapid assessment methods used for health-equity audit: Diabetes mellitus among frail British care-home residents. *Public Health, 120*(11), 1042–1051. https://doi.org/10.1016/j.puhe.2006.06.002

Backett-Milburn, K., Cunningham-Burley, S., & Davis, J. (2003). Contrasting lives, contrasting views? Understandings of health inequalities from children in differing social circumstances. *Social Science & Medicine, 57*, 613–623. https://doi.org/10.1016/S0277-9536(02)00413-6

Baines, D., & Gnanayutham, R. (2018). Rapid ethnography and a knowledge mobilization project: Benefits from bookettes. In P. Armstrong & R. Lowndes (Eds), *Creative Teamwork: Developing Rapid, Site-Switching Ethnography* (pp. 156–170). Oxford University Press.

Barker, J., & Weller, S. (2003). 'Is It Fun?' Developing children centred research methods. *International Journal of Sociology and Social Policy, 23*(1/2), 33–58. https://doi.org/10.1108/01443330310790435

Bauman, A. E., Nelson, D. E., Pratt, M., Matsudo, V., & Schoeppe, S. (2006). Dissemination of physical activity evidence, programs, policies, and surveillance in the international public health arena. *American Journal of Preventive Medicine, 31*(Suppl. 1), S57–S65. https://doi.org/10.1016/j.amepre.2006.06.026

Beebe, J. (1995). Basic concepts and techniques of rapid appraisal. *Human Organization, 54*(1), 42–51. https://doi.org/10.17730/humo.54.1.k84tv883mr2756l3

Beebe, J. (2001). *Rapid Assessment Process: An Introduction*. AltaMira Press.

Beebe, J. (2004). Rapid assessment process. In *Encyclopedia of Social Measurement*. Elsevier.

Beebe, J. (2014). *Rapid Qualitative Inquiry: A Field Guide to Team-Based Assessment* (2nd ed.). Rowman and Littlefield.

Bentley, M., Pelto, G., Straus, W., Schumann, D., Adegbola, C., de la Pena, E., & Huffman, S. L. (1988). Rapid ethnographic assessment: Applications in diarrhea management program. *Social Science and Medicine, 27*(1), 107–116. https://doi.org/10.1016/0277-9536(88)90168-2

Bikker, A., Atherton, H., Brant, H., Porqueddu, T., Campbell, J., Gibson, A., & Ziebland, S. (2017). Conducting a team-based multi-sited focused ethnography in primary care. *BMC Medical Research Methodology, 17*, 139. https://doi.org/10.1186/s12874-017-0422-5

Bjornson-Benson, W. M., Stibolt, T. B., Manske, K. A., Zavela, K. J., Youtsey, D. J., & Buist, A. S. (1993). Monitoring recruitment effectiveness and cost in a clinical trial. *Controlled Clinical Trials, 14*(Suppl. 2), 52S–67S. https://doi.org/10.1016/0197-2456(93)90024-8

Bowen, S., Bottling, I., Graham, I., MacLeod, M., Moissac, de., D, Harlos., & Knox, J. (2019). Experience of health leadership in partnering with university-based researchers

in Canada – A call to 're-imagine' research. *International Journal of Health Policy and Management, 8*(12), 684–699. https://doi.org/10.15171/ijhpm.2019.66
Braun, V., & Clarke, V. (2006). Using thematic analysis in psychology. *Qualitative Research in Psychology, 3*, 77–101. https://doi.org/10.1191/1478088706qp063oa
Brown, D., Hernandez, A., Saint-Jean, G., Evans, S., Tafari, I., Brewster, L.G., & Page, J.B. (2008). A participatory action research pilot study of urban health disparities using rapid assessment response and evaluation. *American Journal of Public Health, 98*(1), 28–38. https://doi.org/10.2105/AJPH.2006.091363
Brown, D. R., Hernández, A., Saint-Jean, G., Evans, S., Tafari, I., Brewster, L. G., . . . Page, J. B. (2008). A participatory action research pilot study of urban health disparities using rapid assessment response and evaluation. *American Journal of Public Health, 98*(1), 28–38.
Chambers, R. (1981). Rapid rural appraisal: Rationale and repertoire. *Public Administration and Development, 1*(2), 95–106.
Chambers, R. (1991). Shortcut and participatory methods for gaining social information for projects. In M. Cernea (Ed.), *Putting People First: Sociological Variables in Rural Development* (pp. 515–537). Oxford University Press/World Bank.
Chambers, R. (1994). Participatory rural appraisal (PRA): Challenges, potentials and paradigm. *World Development, 22*(10), 1437–1454. http://dx.doi.org/10.1016/0305-750x(94)90030-2
Chambers, R. (1994). Participatory rural appraisal (PRA): Analysis of experience. *World Development, 22*(9), 1253–1268. https://doi.org/10.1016/0305-750X(94)90003-5
Chambers, R. (1994a). The origins and practice of participatory rural appraisal. *World Development, 22*(7), 953–969. https://doi.org/10.1016/0305-750X(94)90141-4
Chambers, R. (2008). *Revolutions in Development Inquiry*. Earthscan.
Chambers, R., & Blackburn, J. (1996). *The Power of Participation*. Institute of Development Studies, University of Sussex.
Chesluk, B. J., Bernabeo, E., Reddy, S., Lynn, L., Hess, B., & Odhner, T. (2015). How hospitalists work to pull healthcare teams together. *Journal of Health Organization and Management, 29*(7), 933–947. https://doi.org/10.1108/JHOM-01-2015-0008
Chesluk, B. J., & Holmboe, E. S. (2010). How teams work – or don't – in primary care: A field study on internal medicine practices. *Health Affairs, 29*(5), 874–879. https://doi.org/10.1377/hlthaff.2009.1093
Chowdhury, S. N. M., & Moni, D. (2004). A situation analysis of the menstrual regulation programme in Bangladesh. *Reproductive Health Matters, 12*(Suppl. 24), 95–104. https://doi.org/10.1016/S0968-8080(04)24020-4
Choy, I., Kitto, S., Adu-Aryee, N., & Okrainec, A. (2013). Barriers to the uptake of laparoscopic surgery in a lower-middle-income country. *Surgical Endoscopy, 27*, 4009–4015. https://doi.org/10.1007/s00464-013-3019-z
Colquhoun, H. L., Levac, D., O'Brien, K. K., Straus, S., Tricco, A. C., Perrier, L., & Moher, D. (2014). Scoping reviews: Time for clarity in definition, methods, and reporting. *Journal of Clinical Epidemiology, 67*(12), 1291–1294. https://doi.org/10.1016/j.jclinepi.2014.03.013
Coreil, J., Augustin, A., Holt, E., & Halsey, N. A. (1989). Use of ethnographic research for instrument development in a case-control study of immunization use in Haiti. *International Journal of Epidemiology, 18*(4 Suppl. 2), S33–S37. https://doi.org/10.1093/ije/18.Supplement_2.S33
Crabtree, B., & Miller, W. (1999). *Doing Qualitative Research*. SAGE.
Crivello, G., Camfield, L., & Woodhead, M. (2009). How can children tell us about their wellbeing? Exploring the potential of participatory research approaches within young lives. *Social Indicator Research, 90*, 51–72. https://doi.org/10.1007/s11205-008-9312-x

Culhane-Pera, K. A., Sriphetcharawut, S., Thawsirichuchai, R., Yangyuenkun, W., & Kunstadter, P. (2015, November). Afraid of delivering at the hospital or afraid of delivering at home: A qualitative study of Thai Hmong families' decision-making about maternity services. *Maternal and Child Health Journal, 19*(11), 2384–2392. https://doi.org/10.1007/s10995-015-1757-3

Cupit, C., Mackintosh, N., & Armstrong, N. (2018). Using ethnography to study improving healthcare: Reflections on the 'ethnographic' label. *BMJ Quality & Safety, 27*, 258–260. https://doi.org/10.1136/bmjqs-2017-007599

Curtis, K., Liabo, K., Roberts, H., & Barker, M. (2004). Consulted but not heard: A qualitative study of young people's views of their local health service. *Health Expectations, 7*, 149–156. https://doi.org/10.1111/j.1369-7625.2004.00265.x

Daley, C. M., James, A. S., Filippi, M., Weir, M., Braiuca, S., Kaur, B., & Greiner, K. A. (2012). American Indian community leader and provider views of needs and barriers to colorectal cancer screening. *Journal of Health Disparities Research and Practice, 5*(2), 2. https://doi.org/10.1007/s10900-011-9446-7

Davidoff, F., Dixon-Woods, M., Leviton, L., & Michie, S. (2015). Demystifying theory and its use in improvement. *BMJ Quality & Safety, 24*(3), 228–238.

Denzin, N. K., & Lincoln, Y. S. (1995). Transforming qualitative research methods: Is it a revolution? *Journal of Contemporary Ethnography, 24*(3), 349–358. http://dx.doi.org/10.1177/089124195024003006

Desmond, N., Allen, C., Clift, S., Justine, B., Mzugu, J., Plummer, M., & Ross, D. A. (2005). A typology of groups at risk of HIV/STI in a gold mining town in north-western Tanzania. *Social Science & Medicine, 60*, 1739–1749. https://doi.org/10.1016/j.socscimed.2004.08.027

Driscoll, A., Currey, J., Worrall-Carter, L., & Stewart, S. (2008). Ethical dilemmas of a large national multi-centre study in Australia: Time for some consistency. *Journal of Clinical Nursing, 17*(16), 2212–2220. https://doi.org/10.1111/j.1365-2702.2007.02219.x

Dynes, M. M., Miller, L., Sam, T., Vandi, M. A., Tomczyk, B., & Centers for Disease Control and Prevention. (2015). Perceptions of the risk for Ebola and health facility use among health workers and pregnant and lactating women—Kenema District, Sierra Leone, September 2014. *Morbidity and Mortality Weekly Report, 63*(51), 1226–1227.

Ensign, J., & Bell, M. (2004). Illness experiences of homeless youth. *Qualitative Health Research, 14*(9), 1239–1254. https://doi.org/10.1177/1049732304268795

Ewald, W. (2000). *Secret Games: Collaborative Works With Children, 1969-1999*. Scalo.

Felisberto, E., Freese, E., Natal, S., & Alves, C. K. (2008). A contribution to institutionalized health evaluation: A proposal for self-evaluation. *Cadernos de saude publica, 24*(9), 2091–2102. https://doi.org/10.1590/S0102-311X2008000900015

Finch, H., Lewis, J., & Turley, C. (2003). *Qualitative Research Practice: A Guide for Social Science Students and Researchers* (pp. 170–198). Focus Groups.

Fitch, C., Rhodes, T., & Stimson, G. (2000). Origins of an epidemic: The methodological and political emergence of rapid assessment. *International Journal of Drug Policy, 11*, 63–82. https://doi.org/10.1016/S0955-3959(99)00056-0

Flick, U. (2018). *An Introduction to Qualitative Research*. SAGE.

Freeman, M., deMarrais, K., Preissle, J., Roulston, K., & St. Pierre, E. A. (2007). Standards of evidence in qualitative research: An incitement to discourse. *Educational Researcher, 36*(1), 25–32. https://doi.org/10.3102/0013189X06298009

Gale, N. K., Heath, G., Cameron, E., Rashid, S., & Redwood, S. (2013). Using the framework method for the analysis of qualitiative data in multi-disciplinary health research. *BMC Medical Research Methodology, 13*, 117. https://doi.org/10.1186/1471-2288-13-117

Gale, R. C., Wu, J., Erhardt, T., Bounthavong, M., Reardon, C. M., Damschroder, L. J., & Midboe, A. M. (2019). Comparison of rapid vs in-depth qualitative analytic methods from a process evaluation of academic detailing in the Veterans Health Administration. *Implementation Science, 14*(1), 1–12. http://dx.doi.org/10.1186/s13012-019-0853-y

Garcia, C. M., & Saewyc, E. M. (2007). Perceptions of mental health among recently immigrated Mexican adolescents. *Issues in Mental Health Nursing, 28*(1), 37–54. https://doi.org/10.1080/01612840600996257

Garko, B. (2007). Sexual and family planning practices and needs of people living with HIV/AIDS in Nigeria: A rapid ethnographic assessment. *Annals of African Medicine, 6*(3), 124–127. https://doi.org/10.4103/1596-3519.55721

Garrett, J. L., & Downen, J. (2002). Strengthening rapid assessments in urban areas: Lessons from Bangladesh and Tanzania. *Human Organization, 61*, 314–327.

Gittelsohn, J. (1998). *Rapid Assessment Procedures (RAP): Ethnographic Methods to Investigate Women's Health*. International Nutrition Foundation.

Goepp, J. G., Chin, N. P., Malia, T., & Poordabbagh, A. (2004, October). Planning emergency medical services for children in Bolivia: Part 2-results of a rapid assessment procedure. *Pediatric Emergency Care, 20*(10), 664–670. https://doi.org/10.1097/01.pec.0000142950.58265.15

Goepp, J. G., Meykler, S., Mooney, N. E., Lyon, C., Raso, R., & Julliard, K. (2008, August-September). Provider insights about palliative care barriers and facilitators: Results of a rapid ethnographic assessment. *American Journal of Hospice and Palliative Medicine, 25*(4), 309–314. https://doi.org/10.1177/1049909108319265

Grant, L., Brown, J., Leng, M., Bettega, N., & Murray, S. A. (2011). Palliative care making a difference in rural Uganda, Kenya and Malawi: Three rapid evaluation field studies. *BMC Palliative Care*, 10, 8. https://doi.org/10.1186/1472-684X-10-8

Green, J., & Thorogood, N. (2013). *Qualitative Methods for Health Research*. SAGE.

Guerrero, M., Morrow, R., Calva, J., Ortega-Gallegos, H., Weller, S., Ruiz-Palacios, G., & Morrow, A. L. (1999). Rapid ethnographic assessment of breastfeeding practices in periurban Mexico City. *Bulletin of the World Health Organization, 77*(4), 323–330.

Halme, M., Kourula, A., Lindeman, S., Kallio, G., & Lima-Toivanen, M. (2016). Sustainability innovation at the base of the pyramid through multi-sited rapid ethnography. *Corporate Social Responsibility and Environmental Management, 23*, 113–128. https://doi.org/10.1002/csr.1385

Handwerker, P. (2001). *Quick Ethnography: A Guide to Rapid Multi-Method Research*. Rowman Altamira.

Hargreaves, M. B. (2014). *Rapid Evaluation Approaches for Complex Initiatives*. Mathematical Policy Research.

Harris, K. J., Jerome, N. W., & Fawcett, S. B. (1997). Rapid assessment procedures: A review and critique. *Human Organization, 56*(3), 375–378. https://doi.org/10.17730/humo.56.3.w525025611458003

Harte, J. D., Sheehan, A., Stewart, S. C., & Foureur, M. (2016, April). Childbirth supporters' experiences in a built hospital birth environment. *HERD: Health Environments Research & Design Journal, 9*(3), 135–161. https://doi.org/10.1177/1937586715622006

Herman, E., & Bentley, M. (1993). *Rapid Assessment Procedures (RAP) to Improve the Household Management of Diarrhea*. International Foundation for Developing Countries.

Heywood, P. (1990). W(h)ither rapid (Rural) appraisal techniques in nutrition. Unpublished manuscript, Brisbane.

Higginbottom, G. M. A. (2011). The transitioning experiences of internationally-educated nurses into a Canadian health care system: A focused ethnography. *BMC Nursing, 10*(14), 1–13. https://doi.org/10.1186/1472-6955-10-14

Hildebrand, P. (1979). *Summary of the Sondeo methodology used by ICTA*. Paper presented at the Rapid Rural Appraisal Conference at the Institute of Development Studies, University of Sussex, Sussex, UK.

Hoernke, K., Djellouli, N., Andrews, L., Lewis-Jackson, S., Manby, L., Martin, S., & . . . Vindrola-Padros, C. (2021). Frontline healthcare workers' experiences with personal protective equipment during the COVID-19 pandemic in the UK: A rapid qualitative appraisal. *BMJ open, 11*(1). http://dx.doi.org/10.1136/bmjopen-2020-046199

Holdsworth, L., Safaeinili, N., Winget, M., Lorenz, K., Lough, M., Asch, S., & Malcolm, E. (2020). Adapting rapid assessment procedures for implementation research using a team based approach to analysis: A case example of patient quality and safety interventions in the ICU. *Implementation Science, 15*, 12. https://doi.org/10.1186/s13012-020-0972-5

Hubbard, J. (1994). *Shooting Back From the Reservation*. New Press.

Hundt, G. L., Stuttaford, M., Ngoma, B., & Team, SASPI. (2004, July). The social diagnostics of stroke-like symptoms: Healers, doctors and prophets in Agincourt, Limpopo Province, South Africa. *Journal of Biosocial Science, 36*(4), 433–443. https://doi.org/10.1017/S0021932004006662

Hurtado, E. (1990). Use of rapid anthropological procedures by health personnel in Central America. *Food and Nutrition Bulletin, 12*(4), 1–3. http://dx.doi.org/10.1177/156482659001200416

Hussain, R. S., McGarvey, S. T., & Fruzzetti, L. M. (2015). Partition and poliomyelitis: An investigation of the polio disparity affecting Muslims during India's eradication program. *PLOS ONE, 10*, e0115628. https://doi.org/10.1371/journal.pone.0115628

ICJME. (2021). *Defining the role of authors and contributors*. Retrieved from http://www.icmje.org/recommendations/browse/roles-and-responsibilities/defining-the-role-of-authors-and-contributors.html

Iedema, R., Allen, S., Britton, K., & Hor, S. (2012). Out of the frying pan? Streamlining the ethics review process of multisite qualitative research projects. *Australian Health Review, 37*(2), 137–139. https://doi.org/10.1071/AH11044

Ives, J., Greenfield, S., Parry, J. M., Draper, H., Gratus, C., & Petts, J. (2009). Healthcare workers' attitudes to working during pandemic influenza: A qualitative study. *BMC Public Health, 9*, 56. https://doi.org/10.1186/1471-2458-9-56

Jamal, A., & Crisp, J. (2002). *Real-Time Humanitarian Evaluations: Some Frequently Asked Questions*. UNHCR.

Jayawardena, A., Wijayasinghe, S. R., Tennakoon, D., Cook, T., & Morcuende, J. A. (2013). Early effects of a 'train the trainer' approach to Ponseti method dissemination: A case study of Sri Lanka. *Iowa Orthopedic Journal, 33*, 153–160.

Johnson, G. A. (2011). A child's right to participation: Photovoice as methodology for documenting the experiences of children living in Kenyan orphanages. *Visual Anthropology Review, 27*(2), 141–161. https://doi.org/10.1111/j.1548-7458.2011.01098.x

Johnson, G. A., Pfister, A. E., & Vindrola-Padros, C. (2012). Drawings, photos, and performances: Using visual methods with children. *Visual Anthropology Review, 28*(2), 164–178. https://doi.org/10.1111/j.1548-7458.2012.01122.x

Johnson, G. A., & Vindrola-Padros. C. (2017). Rapid qualitative research methods during complex health emergencies: A systematic review of the literature. *Social Science and Medicine, 189*, 63–75. https://doi.org/10.1016/j.socscimed.2017.07.029

Jones, A. (2004). Involving children and young people as researchers. In V. L. S. Fraser, S. Ding, M. Kellet, & C. Robinson (Eds), *Doing Research With Children and Young People* (pp. 113–131). Sage.

Keith, R., Crosson, J., O'Mailey, A., Cromp, D., & Fries Taylor, E. (2017). Using the consolidated framework for implementation research (CFIR) to produce actionable findings: A rapid-cycle evaluation approach to improving implementation. *Implementation Science, 12,* 15. https://doi.org/10.1186/s13012-017-0550-7

Khangura, S., Konnyu, K., Cushman, R., Grimshaw, J., & Moher, D. (2012). Evidence summaries: The evolution of a rapid review approach. *Systematic Reviews, 1,* 10. https://doi.org/10.1186/2046-4053-1-10

Kilian, C., Salmoni, A., Ward-Griffin, C., & Kloseck, M. (2008). Perceiving falls within a family context: A focused ethnographic approach. *Canadian Journal on Aging/La Revue canadienne du vieillissement, 27*(4), 331–345. http://dx.doi.org/10.3138/cja.27.4.331

Kirsch, H. (1995). The use of rapid assessment procedures: Focus groups and small-scale surveys for community programs. In H. Kirsch (Ed.), *Drug Lessons and Education Programs in Developing Countries*. Transaction Publishers.

Knoblauch, H. (2005). Focused ethnography. *Forum Qualitative Sozialforschung / Forum: Qualitative Social Research, 6*(3), 44. http://nbn-resolving.de/urn:nbn:de:0114-fqs0503440

Koh, Y., Hegney, D. G., & Drury, V. (2011). Comprehensive systematic review of healthcare workers' perceptions of risk and use of coping strategies towards emerging respiratory infectious diseases. *International Journal of Evidence-Based Healthcare, 9,* 403–419. https://doi.org/10.1111/j.1744-1609.2011.00242.x

Kresno, S., Harrison, G., Sutrisna, B., & Reingold, A. (1993). Acute respiratory illnesses in children under five years in Indramayu, West Java, Indonesia: A rapid ethnographic assessment. *Medical Anthropology, 15*(4), 425–434. https://doi.org/10.1080/01459740.1994.9966103

Ladner, S. (2014). *Practical Ethnography: A Guide to Doing Ethnography in the Private Sector.* Left Coast Press.

Landis, J. R., & Koch, G. G. (1977). The measurement of observer agreement for categorical data. *Biometrics, 33,* 159. https://doi.org/10.2307/2529310

Lapan, S., Quartaroli, M. T., & Riemer, F. J. (2011). *Qualitative Research: An Introduction to Methods and Designs.* John Wiley & Sons.

Leininger, M. M. (1985). Ethnography and ethnonursing: Models and modes of qualitative data analysis. In M. Leininger (Ed.), *Qualitative Research Methods in Nursing* (pp. 33–72). Grune & Stratton.

Levac, D., Colquhoun, H., & O'Brien, K. K. (2010). Scoping studies: Advancing the methodology. *Implementation Science, 5,* 69. https://doi.org/10.1186/1748-5908-5-69

Liberati, E. G. (2017). What is the potential of patient shadowing as a patient-centred method? *BMJ Quality and Safety, 26,* 343–346.

Long, A., Scrimshaw, S. C. M., & Hurtado, E. (1988). *Epilepsy Rapid Assessment Procedures (ERAP): Rapid Assessment Procedures for the Evaluation of Epilepsy Specific Beliefs, Attitudes and Behaviours*. Epilepsy Foundation of America.

Lowndes, R., & Armstrong, P. (2018). Fieldnotes: Individual versus team-based rapid ethnography. In R. Lowndes, P. Storm, & M. Szebehely (Eds), *Creative Teamwork* (pp. 81–95). Oxford University Press.

Luttrell, W. (2010). 'A camera is a big responsibility': A lens for analysing children's visual voices. *Visual Studies, 25*(3), 224–237. https://doi.org/10.1080/1472586X.2010.523274

Macdonald, S., Gerbich, C., & von Oswald, M. (2018). No museum is an island: Ethnography beyond methodological containerism. *Museum and Society, 16,* 138–156.

MacQueen, K., McLellan, E., Milstein, K., & Milstein, B. (1998). Codebook development for team-based qualitative analysis. *Cultural Anthropology Methods, 10*(2), 31–36. https://doi.org/10.1177/1525822X9801000n.d.1

Manderson, L., & Aaby, P. (1992a). An epidemic in the field? Rapid assessment procedures and health research. *Social Science and Medicine, 35*(7), 839–850. https://doi.org/10.1016/0277-9536(92)90098-B

Manderson, L., & Aaby, P. (1992b). Can rapid anthropological procedures be applied to tropical diseases? *Health Policy and Planning, 7*(1), 46–55. https://doi.org/10.1093/heapol/7.1.46

Mason, B., Epiphaniou, E., Nanton, V., Donaldson, A., Shipman, C., Daveson, B. A., & Murray, S. A. (2013). Coordination of care for individuals with advanced progressive conditions: A multi-site ethnographic and serial interview study. *British Journal of General Practice, 63*, 580–588.

Maunder, R. G., Lancee, W. J., Mae, R., Vincent, L., Peladeau, N., Beduz, M. A., & Leszcz, M. (2010). Computer-assisted resilience training to prepare healthcare workers for pandemic influenza: A randomized trial of the optimal dose of training. *BMC Health Services Research, 10*, 72. https://doi.org/10.1186/1472-6963-10-72

McElroy, T., Konde-Lule, J., Neema, S., Gitta, S., & Uganda Sustainable Clubfoot Care. (2007, June 15–30). Understanding the barriers to clubfoot treatment adherence in Uganda: A rapid ethnographic study. *Disability and Rehabilitation, 29*(11–12), 845–855. https://doi.org/10.1080/09638280701240102

McMullen, C., Ash, J. S., Sittig, D. F., Bunce, A., Guappone, K., Dykstra, R., & Wright, A. (2011). Rapid assessment of clinical information systems in the healthcare setting: An efficient method for time-pressed evaluation. *Methods of Information in Medicine, 50*(4), 299–307. https://doi.org/10.3414/ME10-01-0042

McNall, M. A., & Foster-Fishman, P. (2007). Methods of rapid evaluation, assessment, and appraisal. *American Journal of Evaluation, 28*(2), 151–168. https://doi.org/10.1177/1098214007300895

McNall, M. A., Welch, V. E., Ruh, K. L., Mildner, C. A., & Soto, T. (2004). The use of rapid-feedback evaluation methods to improve the retention rates of an HIV/AIDS healthcare intervention. *Evaluation and Program Planning, 27*, 287–94. https://doi.org/10.1016/j.evalprogplan.2004.04.003

McNally, N. (2020). *Research leadership – You've got to work at, and beyond, the boundaries*. NIHR blog. https://www.uclhospitals.brc.nihr.ac.uk/latest-blogs/research-leadership-you%E2%80%99ve-got-work-and-beyond-boundaries

Miake-Lye, I., Hempel, S., Shanman, R., & Shekelle, P. (2016). What is an evidence map? A systematic review of published evidence maps and their definitions, methods, and products. *Systematic Reviews, 5*, 28. https://doi.org/10.1186/s13643-016-0204-x

Michie, S. (2020). *Behavioural science must be at the heart of the public health response to Covid-19*. https://blogs.bmj.com/bmj/2020/02/28/behavioural-science-must-be-at-the-heart-of-the-public-health-response-to-covid-19/

Mitchell, L. (2006). Child centered? Thinking critically about children's drawings as a visual research method. *Visual Anthropology Review, 22* (1), 60–73. https://doi.org/10.1525/var.2006.22.1.60

Mitchinson, L., Dowrick, A., Buck, C., Hoernke, K., Martin, S., Vanderslott, S., & Vindrola-Padros, C. (2021). Missing the human connection: A rapid appraisal of healthcare workers' perceptions and experiences of providing palliative care during the COVID-19 pandemic. *Palliative Medicine*, 02692163211004228.

Moher, D., Liberati, A., Tetzlaff, J., & Altman, D. G. (2009). Preferred reporting items for systematic reviews and meta-analyses: The PRISMA statement. *Annals of Internal Medicine, 151*(4), 264–269. https://doi.org/10.7326/0003-4819-151-4-200908180-00135

Moher, D., Schulz, K., Simera, I., & Altman, D. (2010). Guidance for developers of health research reporting guidelines. *PLOS Medicine, 7*(2), 1000217. https://doi.org/10.1371/journal.pmed.1000217

Montgomery, H. (2009). *An Introduction to Childhood: An Anthropological Perspective of Children's Lives*. Wiley-Blackwell.

Morse, J. (1994). *Critical Issues in Qualitative Research Methods*. SAGE.

Mullaney, T., Pettersson, H., Nyholm, T., & Stolterman, E. (2012, December). Thinking beyond the cure: A case for human-centered design in cancer care. *International Journal of Design, 6*(3), www.ijdesign.org/index.php/IJDesign/article/view/1076

Munday, D., Haraldsdottir, E., Manak, M., Thyle, A., & Ratcliff, C. M. (2018). Rural palliative care in North India: Rapid evaluation of a program using a realist mixed method approach. *Indian Journal of Palliative Care, 24*(1), 3–8.

Munoz-Plaza, C., Parry, C., Hahn, E., Tang, T., Nguyen, H., Gould, M., & Sharp, A. (2016). Integrating qualitative research methods into care improvement efforts within a learning health system: Addressing antibiotic overuse. *Health Research Policy and Systems, 14*, 63. https://doi.org/10.1186/s12961-016-0122-3

Murray, J. K., DiStefano, A., Yang, J., & Wood, M. (2016, September–October). Displacement and HIV: Factors influencing antiretroviral therapy use by ethnic Shan migrants in Northern Thailand. *The Journal of the Association of Nurses in AIDS Care, 27*(5), 709. https://doi.org/10.1016/j.jana.2016.04.006

Neal, J., Neal, Z., VanDyke, E., & Kornbluh, M. (2015). Expediting the analysis of qualitative data in evaluation: A procedure for the rapid identification of themes from audio recordings (RITA). *American Journal of Evaluation, 36*(1), 118–132. https://doi.org/10.1177/1098214014536601

Needle, R. H., Trotter, R. T., Singer, M., Bates, C., Bryan Page, J., Metzger, D., & Marcelin, L. H. (2003, June). Rapid assessment of the HIV/AIDS crisis in racial and ethnic minority communities: An approach for timely community interventions. *American Journal of Public Health, 93*(6), 970–979. https://doi.org/10.2105/AJPH.93.6.970

Nowell, L. S., Norris, J. M., White, D. E., & Moules, N. J. (2017). Thematic analysis: Striving to meet the trustworthiness criteria. *International Journal of Qualitative Methods, 16*(1), 1–13. https://doi.org/10.1177/1609406917733847

Nunns, H. (2009). Responding to the demand for quicker evaluation findings. *Social Policy Journal of New Zealand, 34*, 89–99.

Pace, R., Pluye, P., & Bartlett, G. (2012). Testing the reliability and efficiency of the pilot mixed methods appraisal tool (MMAT) for systematic mixed studies review. *International Journal of Nursing Studies, 49*(1), 47–53. https://doi.org/10.1016/j.ijnurstu.2011.07.002

Palinkas, L., & Zatzick, D. (2019). Rapid assessment procedure informed clinical ethnography (RAPICE) in pragmatic clinical trials of mental health service implementation: Methods and applied case study. *Administration and Policy in Mental Health and Mental Health Services Research, 46*, 255–270. https://doi.org/10.1007/s10488-018-0909-3

Patmon, F., Gee, P., Rylee, T., & Readdy, N. (2016). Using interactive patient engagement technology in clinical practice: A qualitative assessment of nurses' perceptions. *Journal of Medical Internet Research, 18*(11), 30–42. https://doi.org/10.2196/jmir.5667

Pearson, R. (1989). Rapid assessment procedures are changing the way UNICEF evaluates its projects. *Hygie, 8*(4), 23–25.

Pearson, R., & Kessler, S. (1992). Rapid assessment methodology for evaluation by UNICEF. In N. Scrimshaw & R. Gleason (Eds), *Rapid Assessment Methodologies: Qualitative Methodologies for Planning and Evaluation of Health Related Programs*. International Nutrition Foundation for Developing Countries (INFDC).

Pelander, T., Lehtonen, K., & Leino-Kilpi, H. (2007). Children in the hospital: Elements of quality in drawings. *Journal of Pediatric Nursing, 22*(4), 333–341. https://doi.org/10.1016/j.pedn.2007.06.004

Pfister, A. E., Vindrola-Padros, C., & Johnson, G. A. (2015). Together, we can show you: Using participant-generated visual data in collaborative research. *Collaborative Anthropologies, 7*(1), 26–49. https://doi.org/10.1353/cla.2014.0005

Pink, S., & Morgan, J. (2013). Short term ethnography: Intense routes to knowing. *Symbolic Interactionism, 36*(3), 351–361. https://doi.org/10.1002/symb.66

Polito, C., Cribbs, S., Martin, G., O'Keefe, T., Herr, D., Rice, T., & Sevransky, J. (2014). Navigating the institutional review board approval process in a multicentre observational critical care study. *Critical Care Medicine, 42*(5), 1105–1109. https://doi.org/10.1097/CCM.0000000000000133

Popay, J., Rogers, A., & Williams, G. (1998). Rationale and standards for the systematic review of qualitative literature in health services research. *Qualitative Health Research, 8*(3), 341–351. https://doi.org/10.1177/104973239800800305

Rankl, F., Johnson, G., & Vindrola-Padros, C. (2021). Examining what we know in relation to how we know it: A team-based reflexivity model for rapid qualitative health research. *Qualitative Health Research*. https://doi.org/10.1177/1049732321998062

Raven, J., Wurie, H., & Witter, S. (2018). Health workers' experiences of coping with the Ebola epidemic in Sierra Leone's health system: A qualitative study. *BMC Health Services Research, 18*, 251. https://doi.org/10.1186/s12913-018-3072-3

Regenold, N., & Vindrola-Padros, C. (2021). Gender Matters: A Gender Analysis of Healthcare Workers' Experiences during the First COVID-19 Pandemic Peak in England. *Social Sciences, 10*(2), 43. http://dx.doi.org/10.3390/socsci10020043

Rifkin, S. (1992). Rapid appraisals for health: An overview. *Rapid Rural Appraisal Notes, 16*, 7–12.

Ritchie, J., Lewis, J., & Ellam, G. (2004). Designing and selecting samples. In J. Ritchie & J. Lewis (Eds.), *Qualitative Research Practice: A Guide for Social Science Students and Researchers*. SAGE.

Roberts, H. (2000). Listening to children: And hearing them. In P. Christensen & A. James (Eds.), *Research with Children: Perspectives and Practices* (pp. 225–240). Falmer Press.

Rowa-Dewar, N., Ager, W., Ryan, K., Hargan, I., Hubbard, G., & Kearney, N. (2008). Using a rapid appraisal approach in a nationwide, multisite public involvement study in Scotland. *Qualitative Health Research, 18*(6), 863–869. https://doi.org/10.1177/1049732308318735

Saleem, J. J., Plew, W. R., Speir, R. C., Herout, J., Wilck, N. R., & Ryan, D. M. (2015, July). Understanding barriers and facilitators to the use of clinical information systems for intensive care units and anesthesia record keeping: A rapid ethnography. *International Journal of Medical Informatics, 84*(7), 500–511. https://doi.org/10.1016/j.ijmedinf.2015.03.006

San Juan, N. V., Aceituno, D., Djellouli, N., Sumray, K., Regenold, N., Syversen, A., . . . Vindrola-Padros, C. (2021). Mental health and well-being of healthcare workers during the COVID-19 pandemic in the UK: Contrasting guidelines with experiences in practice. *BJPsych Open, 7*(1). http://dx.doi.org/10.1192/bjo.2020.148

Sandison, P. (2003). *Desk Review of Real-Time Evaluation Experience*. United Nations Children's Fund.

Sangaramoorthy, T., & Kroeger, K. (2020). *Rapid Ethnographic Assessments: A Practical Approach and Toolkit for Collaborative Community Research*. Routledge.

Schneeweiss, S., Shrank, W. H., Ruhl, M., & Maclure, M. (2015). Decision-making aligned with rapid-cycle evaluation in health care. *International Journal of Technology Assessment in Health Care, 31*, 214–222. https://doi.org/10.1017/S0266462315000410

Schwitters, A., Lederer, P., Zilversmit, L., Gudo, P. S., Ramiro, I., & Cumba, L. (2015, March 5). Barriers to health care in rural Mozambique: A rapid ethnographic assessment of planned mobile health clinics for ART. *Global Health: Science and Practice, 3*(1), 109–116. https://doi.org/10.9745/GHSP-D-14-00145

Scott, K., McMahon, S., Yumkella, F., Diaz, T., & George, A. (2014, May). Navigating multiple options and social relationships in plural health systems: A qualitative study exploring healthcare seeking for sick children in Sierra Leone. *Health Policy Plan, 29*(3), 292–301. https://doi.org/10.1093/heapol/czt016

Scrimshaw, S., Carballo, M., Ramos, L., & Blair, B. (1991). The AIDS rapid anthropological assessment procedures: A tool for health education planning and evaluation. *Health Education Quarterly, 18*(1), 111–123. https://doi.org/10.1177/109019819101800111

Scrimshaw, S., & Hurtado, E. (1984). Field guide for the study of health-seeking behaviour at the household level. *Food and Nutrition Bulletin, 6*(2), 27–45. https://doi.org/10.1177/156482658400600211

Scrimshaw, S., & Hurtado, E. (1987). *Rapid Assessment Procedures for Nutrition and Primary Health Care. Anthropological Approaches to Improving Programme Effectiveness*. The United Nations University.

Shaw, B., Amouzou, A., Miller, N. P., Tafesse, M., Bryce, J., & Surkan, P. J. (2016). Access to integrated community case management of childhood illnesses services in rural Ethiopia: A qualitative study of the perspectives and experiences of caregivers. *Health Policy Plan, 31*(5), 656–666. https://doi.org/10.1093/heapol/czv115

Shrank, W. (2013). The Center for Medicare and Medicaid innovation's blueprint for rapid-cycle evaluation of new care and payment models. *Health Affairs, 32*(4), 807–812. https://doi.org/10.1377/hlthaff.2013.0216

Singleton, G., Dowrick, A., Manby, L., Fillmore, H., Syversen, A., Lewis-Jackson, S., . . . Vindrola-Padros, C. (2021, under review). *UK health care workers' experiences of major system change in elective surgery during the COVID-19 pandemic: Reflections on rapid service adaptation*. https://www.medrxiv.org/content/10.1101/2021.04.14.21255415v1

Skårås, M. (2018). Focused ethnographic research on teaching and learning in conflict zones: History education in South Sudan. *Forum for Development Studies, 45*(2), 217–238. https://doi.org/10.1080/08039410.2016.1202316

Skillman, M., Cross-Barnet, C., Friedman, R., Rotondo, C., Ruiz, S., & Moiduddin, A. (2019). A framework for rigorous qualitative research as a component of mixed method rapid-cycle evaluation. *Qualitative Health Research, 29*(2), 279–289. https://doi.org/10.1177/1049732318795675

Smith, J., & Firth, J. (2011). Qualitative data analysis: The framework approach. *Nurse Researcher, 18*(2), 52–62. https://doi.org/10.7748/nr2011.01.18.2.52.c8284

Snape, D., & Spencer, L. (2004). Foundations of qualitative research. In J. Ritchie & J. Lewis (Eds.), *Qualitative Research Practice: A Guide for Social Science Students and Researchers* (pp. 1–23). SAGE.

Spradley, J. (1980). *Participant Observation*. New York: Holt, Rinehart, & Winston.

Stimson, G., Fitch, C., & Rhodes, T. (1997). *The Guide on Rapid Assessment Methods for Drug Injecting*. World Health Organization Programme on Substance Abuse.

Storesund, A., & McMurray, A. (2009). Quality of practice in an intensive care unit (ICU): A mini-ethnographic case study. *Intensive and Critical Care Nursing, 25*, 120–127. https://doi.org/10.1016/j.iccn.2009.02.001

Tattersall, C., & Vernon, S. (2007). Mind mapping as a tool in qualitative research. *Nursing Times, 103*(26), 32–33.

Taylor, B., Henshall, C., Kenyon, S., Litchfield, I., & Greenfield, S. (2018). Can rapid approaches to qualitative analysis deliver timely, valid findings to clinical leaders? A mixed methods study comparing rapid and thematic analysis. *BMJ Open, 8*(10), e019993. http://dx.doi.org/10.1136/bmjopen-2017-019993

Taylor, S., Bogdan, R., & DeVault, M. (2015). *Introduction to Qualitative Research Methods: A Guidebook and Resource*. John Wiley and Sons.

Thomas, N., & O'Kane, C. (1998). The ethics of participatory research with children. *Children & Society, 12*, 336–348. https://doi.org/10.1111/j.1099-0860.1998.tb00090.x

Thomas, N., & O'Kane, C. (2000). Discovering what children think: Connections between research and practice. *British Journal of Social Work, 30*, 819–835. https://doi.org/10.1093/bjsw/30.6.819

Tong, A., Sainsbury, P., & Craig, J. (2007). Consolidated criteria for reporting qualitative research (COREQ): A 32-item checklist for interviews and focus groups. *International Journal for Quality in Health Care, 19*, 349–357. https://doi.org/10.1093/intqhc/mzm042

Tricco, A. C., Langlois, E. V., & Straus, S. E. (2017). *Rapid Reviews to Strengthen Health Policy and Systems: A Practical Guide*. World Health Organization, Alliance for Health Policy and Systems Research. www.who.int/alliance-hpsr/resources/publications/rapid-review-guide/en

Tricco, A. C., Lillie, E., Zarin, W., O'Brien, K. K., Colquhoun, H., Levac, D., & Hempel, S. (2018). PRISMA extension for scoping reviews (PRISMA-ScR): Checklist and explanation. *Annals of Internal Medicine, 169*(7), 467–473. https://doi.org/10.7326/M18-0850

Trotter, R. T., Needle, R. H., Goosby, E., Bates, C., & Singer, M. (2001). A methodological model for rapid assessment, response, and evaluation: The RARE program in public health. *Field Methods, 13*(2), 137–159. https://doi.org/10.1177/1525822X0101300202

Trotter, R. T., & Singer, M. (2005). Rapid assessment strategies for public health: Promise and problems. In E. Trickett & W. Pequegnat (Eds), *Community Intervention and AIDS*. Oxford University Press.

UNHCR (2002). Real-time evaluations. *Forced Migration Review, 14*, 43.

Utarini, A., Winkvist, A., & Pelto, G. (2001). Appraising studies in health using rapid assessment procedures (RAP): Eleven critical criteria. *Human Organization, 60*(4), 390–400.

Vincent, N., Allsop, S., & Shoobridge, J. (2000). The use of rapid assessment methodology (RAM) for investigating illicit drug use: A South Australian experience. *Drug and Alcohol Review, 19*, 419–426. https://doi.org/10.1080/713659426

Vindrola-Padros, C. (2012). The everyday lives of children with cancer in Argentina: Going beyond the disease and treatment. *Children and Society, 26*(6), 430–442. https://doi.org/10.1111/j.1099-0860.2011.00369.x

Vindrola-Padros, C. (2020). *Rapid Ethnographies: A Practical Guide*. University of Cambridge Press.

Vindrola-Padros, C., Andrews, L., Dowrick, A., Djellouli, N., Fillmore, H., Gonzalez, E. B., . . . Johnson, G. (2020a). Perceptions and experiences of healthcare workers during the COVID-19 pandemic in the UK. *BMJ Open, 10*(11), e040503. http://dx.doi.org/10.1136/bmjopen-2020-040503

Vindrola-Padros, C., Brage, E., & Johnson, G. A. (2021). Rapid, Responsive, and Relevant? A Systematic Review of Rapid Evaluations in Health Care. *American Journal of Evaluation, 42*(1), 13–27.

Vindrola-Padros, C., Chisnall, G., Cooper, S., Dowrick, A., Djellouli, N., Symmons, S. M., & Johnson, G. A. (2020b). Carrying out rapid qualitative research during a pandemic: Emerging lessons from COVID-19. *Qualitative Health Research, 30*(14), 2192–2204. https://doi.org/10.1177/1049732320951526

Vindrola-Padros, C., & Johnson, G. A. (2020). Rapid techniques in qualitative research: A critical review of the literature. *Qualitative Health Research, 30*(10), 1596–1604. https://doi.org/10.1177/1049732320921835

Vindrola-Padros, C., & Vindrola-Padros, B. (2018). Quick and dirty? A systematic review of the use of rapid ethnographies in healthcare organisation and delivery. *BMJ Quality & Safety, 27*, 321–330. https://doi.org/10.1136/bmjqs-2017-007226

Vougioukalou, S., Boaz, A., Gager, M., & Locock, L. (2019). The contribution of ethnography to the evaluation of quality improvement in hospital settings: Reflections on observing co-design in intensive care units and lung cancer pathways in the UK. *Anthropology & Medicine, 26*(1), 18–32. https://doi.org/10.1080/13648470.2018.1507104

Wall, S. (2015). Focused ethnography: A methodological adaptation for social research in emerging contexts [40 paragraphs]. *Forum Qualitative Sozialforschung/Forum: Qualitative Social Research, 16*(1), Art. 1. http://nbn-resolving.de/urn:nbn:de:0114-fqs150111

Wang, C. (1999). A participatory action research strategy applied to women's health. *Journal of Women's Health, 8*, 85–192. https://doi.org/10.1089/jwh.1999.8.185

Watkins, D. (2017). Rapid and rigorous qualitative data analysis: The 'RADaR' technique for applied research. *International Journal of Qualitative Methods, 16*, 1–9. https://doi.org/10.1177/1609406917712131

Weller, S., & Romney, A. (1988). *Systematic Data Collection*. SAGE.

Werner, O., & Schoepfle, G. M. (1987). *Systematic Fieldwork* (Vol. 1B2). Sage Publications.

Whiteford, L., & Vindrola-Padros, C. (2015). *Community Participatory Involvement: A Sustainable Model for Global Public Health*. Routledge.

Williams, H. A., Kachur, S. P., Nalwamba, N. C., Hightower, A., Simoonga, C., & Mphande, P. C. (1999). A community perspective on the efficacy of malaria treatment options for children in Lundazi District, Zambia. *Tropical Medicine & International Health, 4*(10), 641–652. http://dx.doi.org/10.1046/j.1365-3156.1999.00471.x

Wilson, P. M., Petticrew, M., Calnan, M. W., & Nazareth, I. (2010). Does dissemination extend beyond publication: A survey of a cross section of public funded research in the UK. *Implementation Science, 5*, 61. https://doi.org/10.1186/1748-5908-5-61

Wood, V. J., Vindrola, C., Swart, N., McIntosh, M., Crowe, S., Morris, S., & Fulop, N. (2018). One to one specialling and sitters in acute care hospitals: A scoping review. *International Journal of Nursing Studies, 84*, 61–77. https://doi.org/10.1016/j.ijnurstu.2018.04.018

Wright, A., Sittig, D. F., Ash, J. S., Erickson, J. L., Hickman, T. T., Paterno, M., & Middleton, B. (2015, November). Lessons learned from implementing service-oriented clinical decision support at four sites: A qualitative study. *International Journal of Medical Informatics, 84*(11), 901–911. https://doi.org/10.1016/j.ijmedinf.2015.08.008

Young, L., & Barret, H. (2001). Adapting visual methods: Action research with Kamala street children. *Area, 33*(2), 141–152. https://doi.org/10.1111/1475-4762.00017

Zakocs, R., Hill, J. A., Brown, P., Wheaton, J., & Freire, K. E. (2015). The data-to-action framework: A rapid program improvement process. *Health Education & Behavior: The Official Publication of the Society for Public Health Education, 42*(4), 471–479. https://doi.org/10.1177/1090198115595010

Zarinpoush, F., Sychowski, S. V., & Sperling. J. (2007). *Effective Knowledge Transfer and Exchange: A Framework*. Imagine Canada.

Zatzick, D., Rivera, F., Jurkovich, G., Russo, J., Trusz, S. G., Wang, J., & Katon, W. (2011). Enhancing the population impact of collaborative care interventions: Mixed method development and implementation of stepped care targeting posttraumatic stress disorder and related comorbidities after acute trauma. *General Hospital Psychiatry, 33*, 123–134. https://doi.org/10.1016/j.genhosppsych.2011.01.001

INDEX